# The Right to Try

# The Right to Try

How the Federal Government
Prevents Americans from Getting the
Lifesaving Treatments They Need

———

# Darcy Olsen

HARPER

NEW YORK · LONDON · TORONTO · SYDNEY

A hardcover edition of this book was published in 2015 by HarperCollins Publishers.

THE RIGHT TO TRY. Copyright © 2017 by Darcy Olsen. All rights reserved. Printed in the United States of America. No part of this book may be used or reproduced in any manner whatsoever without written permission except in the case of brief quotations embodied in critical articles and reviews. For information, address HarperCollins Publishers, 195 Broadway, New York, NY 10007.

HarperCollins books may be purchased for educational, business, or sales promotional use. For information, please e-mail the Special Markets Department at SPsales@harpercollins.com.

FIRST HARPER PAPERBACKS EDITION PUBLISHED 2017.

Designed by Renato Stanisic

Library of Congress Cataloging-in-Publication Data has been applied for.

ISBN 978-0-06-240753-5 (pbk.)

17 18 19 20 21   OV/LSC   10 9 8 7 6 5 4 3 2 1

To my father, Rick Olsen, and his brother Kenny

# Contents

_____

# Introduction

———

*"Marco!"*

*"Polo!"*

Ted Harada dived under the glistening water of his backyard pool and swam toward the giggling voices of his three children, who scattered to escape their father's grasp.

But as soon as he was underwater, Ted felt his lungs tighten. A sudden drowning sensation overcame him. When he broke through the surface, he was gasping for air.

He looked back. He had swum only a few feet. What on earth was going on? He had played this game with his kids hundreds of times. Why was he having trouble breathing?

His wife, Michelle, called out, "Ted, are you all right?"

"Yeah, I'm fine," Ted told her.

But Ted was not fine. It was late summer of 2009 and Ted had felt himself getting fatigued more easily of late. Despite the fact that he was biking and exercising regularly, he found he was increasingly out of breath. But nothing like this. This was different.

He got out of the pool, dried off, and tried to put the incident out of his mind.

A few months later, Ted went on a fall hike with a group of friends in the north Georgia mountains. It was just a mile-long journey and not a particularly steep incline. Ted had done hikes like this dozens of times before.

But after a few minutes, his left leg started shaking uncontrollably. He stopped.

His friends came back and needled him.

"Come on, Ted, suck it up," they said.

"No, guys, I can't go any farther," he told them, bent over trying to calm his leg and catch his breath.

They became concerned.

"Ted, are you okay?" they asked.

"Honestly, I don't know."

His leg felt like rubber. He had not told anyone about the incident at the pool.

"I guess it's just not my day," Ted finally told them. "You guys go ahead."

They figured he was coming down with something and helped him back to the car. Ted insisted they finish the climb and so they left him there.

Alone in the car, he felt frustrated, scared, and lost.

"What's happening to me?" he thought.

When he got home, he told Michelle what had happened. "Ted, you need to go to a doctor and get checked out," she said. He promised that he would. But, like most people, he put it off. Weeks went by, and Michelle kept reminding him. So finally he gave in and made an appointment to see a doctor at his local family practice.

After examining him, the doctor said Ted probably had asthma and prescribed an inhaler. He used it for a month or so, but it had no effect.

As fall turned into winter, his bouts of breathlessness grew worse. One day, while walking the dog, Ted noticed that he was walking with a limp. His left leg was not keeping up with his right. So he went to an orthopedist he had known for several years, Dr. Vincent Smith, to check out his left leg.

Dr. Smith confirmed the weakness in the leg, and took X-rays and an MRI. They came back all clear.

"You might have a pinched nerve in your back," Dr. Smith told Ted. "Let's get you to a neurosurgeon."

When the neurosurgeon examined Ted, she found that he had weakness not only in his left leg, but also in his left arm and left hand. She told Ted to come to the hospital the next day for an MRI of his brain and spinal cord.

"Maybe I'll need surgery," Ted thought.

When he arrived, the neurosurgeon also conducted an MRA—a magnetic resonance angiogram—checking the blood vessels in Ted's brain to see if he's had a stroke. But all the tests came back clear. Nothing explained Ted's symptoms.

The neurosurgeon handed Ted a disk with all his test data on it and told him, "Ted, there's definitely something wrong, but there's nothing I can do. You need to go see a neurologist."

Now Ted was really starting to get desperate. He called the orthopedist, Dr. Smith, and asked if he could come back and see him that day. Sensing the panic in Ted's voice, Dr. Smith found an opening for Ted that afternoon.

When he arrived at the doctor's office, Ted told him, "You told me to go to a neurosurgeon and she says she can't see anything, and that I need to go see a neurologist. What's going on?" Dr. Smith popped the disk into his computer and spent forty-five minutes going through all the images with Ted, showing him that everything was as it should be.

"I'm gonna be honest, Ted," Dr. Smith told him. "Whatever is going on with you is not common. You need to go up to Emory University and see someone who is used to treating zebras. We only see horses here. You need a zebra doctor."

"A zebra doctor?" Ted thought.

Dr. Smith gave Ted the number for Emory's Department of Neurology. Ted got into his car and called Emory from right there in the parking lot. It was March, but the nurse who answered the phone told him their next opening was not until August.

"I can't wait five months to find out what is wrong with me," Ted told her.

She suggested he contact Dr. David Williams at the Peachtree Neurological Clinic. Williams had done a fellowship at Emory and was highly recommended. Ted called and made an appointment.

A few days later, Dr. Williams saw Ted. He reviewed the MRIs and the tests the other doctors had performed. He examined Ted, testing the strength of his legs, arms, and hands. He told Ted to get dressed while he went to the other room to review the MRIs again.

When he returned, Ted's frustration bubbled up to the surface.

"Doc, just lay it out for me," Ted pleaded. "I've spent eight months getting bounced around from doctor to doctor, and every doctor says there's something wrong but they don't know what's wrong. I don't think I'm crazy. This isn't just in my head. What's happening to me?"

"No, it's not in your head," Dr. Williams told him. "You potentially have a very serious problem. I need to do some more tests. I'd like you to come in Thursday and I want you to bring your wife with you."

Bring his wife? Ted had never had a doctor tell him to bring his wife to an appointment before.

"Why do I need to bring my wife with me?" Ted asked. "Please, just tell me what you think is going on."

Dr. Williams told Ted that he could be suffering from motor neuron disease—a disorder that affects the cells that control muscle movement. He needed to do another test to be sure.

When Ted returned with Michelle on Thursday, Dr. Williams administered an EMG, or electromyogram—a test in which the doctor sticks needles into the muscles and measures the nerve waves from the spinal cord to the muscles. When the results came back, they confirmed

Ted's worst fears. Dr. Williams found abnormalities in Ted's foot, left calf, left thigh, and left hand.

"I'm sorry" Dr. Williams told him, "but I am 80 to 90 percent sure you have ALS—Lou Gehrig's disease. It's a fatal disease."

"How long have I got?" Ted asked him.

"I'm not looking to scare you," Dr. Williams told him. "Some people live two to five years. Others are slow progressors, and live eight to ten years." He wrote Ted a prescription for a medication called Rilutek.

"It's the only approved drug to treat ALS," Dr. Williams told him. "They've shown it can extend your life two to four months on average."

Ted's heart sank. Two to four months? That's it?

Dr. Williams told Ted that he should never accept a terminal diagnosis like this without getting a second opinion and gave him several choices. He could get Ted into Emory University's ALS center, where he had done a fellowship under its director, Dr. Jonathan Glass. He mentioned in passing that Emory was doing some interesting clinical trials, including a stem-cell trial. But he also said that Ted should not feel pressured to go to Emory—he could also get him into the Mayo Clinic in Jacksonville or into some other ALS centers.

Ted decided on Emory.

It would prove to be a fateful choice.

A few weeks later, Ted found himself sitting on an examining table at the Emory University ALS clinic. Emory is a teaching hospital, so when Dr. Glass walked in he was with a group of medical students. They began examining Ted.

"I'm in an episode of *House*," Ted thought.

After the exam was over, Dr. Glass asked, "So what did Dr. Williams tell you?"

"He said he was pretty sure I had ALS," Ted replied.

Dr. Glass's demeanor changed. He put his hand on Ted's knee.

"I'm sorry to tell you this, but you do have ALS. You need to know that there's nothing you did to get it and nothing you could have done to avoid getting it. And I have to apologize too, because my career has been devoted to finding a cure, but right now I don't have a cure for you. It's 100 percent fatal."

He told Ted that 80 percent of people with ALS die within five years of diagnosis.

Up until that moment, Ted had been holding on to hope. But now his world shattered. Here he was in the doctor's office and, instead of discussing treatment options, Dr. Glass was explaining that he needed a will and to get his affairs in order.

Ted had received a death sentence.

Following his diagnosis, Ted went home. One of his friends lent him and Michelle his weekend home in the mountains so they could get away and be alone together. Sitting on the front porch, they finally broke down. Ted told her he was sorry—for letting her down and letting their kids down. Nonsense, she told him, her eyes welling with tears, he had nothing to be sorry about. He and Michelle cried in each other's arms, as all the bottled-up emotions finally came pouring out.

It was one of the hardest nights of Ted's life.

"But the next day, the sun rose," Ted says, "and so did I."

Over breakfast, he told Michelle he loved her and that the night before had been cathartic. "We needed that," he said, "But I don't want to do that every day. Look, this disease is going to take me. But right now, I'm still alive. I don't want to be mourned while I'm alive."

Ted also decided that he was not going down without a fight. He began to study ALS. What he found was not encouraging. ALS is a cruel disease. It causes the motor neurons inside your spinal cord to selectively die. A motor neuron sends wires out to the muscles with signals instructing them to move. When the motor neurons die, the wires that go out to the muscles degenerate or die. When the wires die, the signals stop. When the signals stop, the muscles begin to atrophy and die. And when the muscles that control swallowing and breathing die, you die.

The one part of the body not affected in most cases is cognition—which means that patients are aware of everything that is happening to them every step of the way.

It is a horrific way to go.

Ted's condition began to rapidly deteriorate. A man who loved to wrestle on the floor with his children now could barely make it up the stairs to kiss them good night. He could walk only short distances with the help of a cane. Simple tasks, like getting the mail, became unbearable chores.

As his symptoms grew worse, Ted had to quit his job as the district manager at a shredding company.

Eventually, his hands became so weak that he could not even open a Ziploc bag.

Ted Harada was dying.

On October 20, 2012, two years after his diagnosis, Ted bent over and tied the laces on his running shoes. He stood up, without the help of a cane, and walked confidently to the starting line to begin Atlanta's two-and-a-half mile "Walk to Defeat ALS."

He completed the full course without any difficulty whatsoever. His left leg kept pace with his right. He had no shortness of breath.

Not only was Ted walking again; he was back in the family pool playing Marco Polo with his kids. At night, he bounded up the stairs to tuck them into bed. He was biking, hiking, and walking the dog just like he used to. His lungs felt strong and his grip had returned.

He could go most days without thinking he had ALS.

His transformation was nothing short of miraculous. No one in recorded history had ever gotten better after a diagnosis of ALS.

*No one.*

But Ted Harada was getting better.

Like Lazarus of the Bible, who rose from the dead, Ted had experienced a modern-day resurrection.

When Dr. Williams and Dr. Glass first diagnosed Ted, they were clear that there was no cure for ALS. But that was not good enough for Ted. If he was going to die, so be it—but he was going to fight this disease until it stole his very last breath.

As he began to research emerging treatments, he found that his doctors were right. Every drug being tried was failing. Nothing slowed the advance of the disease. And certainly nothing reversed it.

That was about to change.

No one can call an ALS diagnosis a blessing, but Ted Harada was blessed to have been diagnosed at the right place, at the right time, by the right doctors. Ted lived near Atlanta, which just happens to be home to one of the nation's leading centers for ALS research. And his diagnosis came just as an Emory-led team of medical researchers was about to shock the world with perhaps the biggest breakthrough ever in the treatment of ALS.

Surgeons at Emory were getting ready to try an unprecedented new procedure in which they would inject stem cells into the diseased areas of the spinal cord, where the pools of motor neurons affected by ALS are located. The hope was that the inserted cells would repair and replace the damaged and diseased cells and thus slow or stop or perhaps even reverse the degeneration of the motor neurons.

The surgery—which had been pioneered by Dr. Nick Boulis of Emory University and a Bethesda, Maryland, pharmaceutical firm called Neuralstem—was revolutionary. Doctors were not simply injecting the cells into the spinal cavity or the spinal fluid. They planned to open up the spinal cord itself and transplant the cells directly into the gray matter of the spinal cord—beyond the blood-brain barrier.

Intraspinal surgery like this had never been tried before. It was incredibly risky. One mistake, even the slightest movement, could cause irreparable damage to the spinal nerves. The patient could be instantly paralyzed, or worse.

The experimental surgery was being performed only at Emory, which happened to be just forty-five minutes from Ted Harada's home.

When Ted learned about the surgery, he told Dr. Glass and his team, "I want to do this trial." It had been in the back of his head ever since Dr. Williams had mentioned it in passing the day he was first diagnosed.

But it turned out getting into the trial was not so easy. The researchers at Emory told Ted that they were not recruiting for the trial at that moment. Perhaps he might want to look at other options? "No," Ted told them. He wanted to wait to be in the stem-cell trial. He asked them to tell him as soon as they began recruiting again.

Every week he emailed Crystal Kelly, one of the clinical research coordinators, reminding her that he wanted to be considered. Every week the answer was the same: We're not recruiting yet.

Finally, after a month of persistent nagging, they told Ted that they were recruiting again and he should come in for a screening to see if he qualified.

The day Ted arrived at Emory, there was a TV crew from Fox 5 news there to film another patient who was undergoing the experimental surgery that day.

Ted took it as a sign.

When Ted was finally accepted into the trial, Dr. Glass and his team tried to temper his hopes. They explained that the procedure was in phase I safety trials. The objective was not to help Ted, but to show that the procedure itself would not kill him.

Ted told them he understood. He had made peace with his diagnosis.

"If this is what the cutting edge is, then you need people to move the ball. You need people to man the spaceships. Let me be that person," he said.

When he was accepted into the trial, his parents and his in-laws were elated. It was the first sign of hope they had had since learning of his terminal diagnosis. Ted had to explain to them that the surgery was only to help others.

Yes, they said, but it *could* help you.

"No," he insisted, "it can't. They told me it's not going to help me."

But in the back of his mind, he held the smallest bit of hope. He looked at it like buying a lottery ticket. "You don't win when you buy a lottery ticket," Ted thought, "but you know that saying 'You can't win if you don't buy a ticket'? Well, this was my ticket."

Dr. Glass and his colleagues were blunt about the danger he faced. The surgery had been tried only a few times before. It could paralyze him. It could kill him. Ted signed a fifteen-page consent form acknowledging he understood all the risks. Emory then videotaped him and Michelle, explaining to them on camera that this was a safety study that was designed not to benefit him, but for the benefit of future patients down the line.

At one point Ted turned to Dr. Glass and said, "Look, I get it. But I feel like I have a moral obligation for those people who come after me to do what I can."

Dr. Glass stopped him cold.

"You have no obligation to do this, Ted," he said.

"Look, I get the legalese," Ted told him. "I am not suggesting that you are telling me I have an obligation. I am telling you morally I feel like I have a duty to do this for my fellow man."

If he could not save himself, Ted figured, perhaps he could help save others.

And who knows, he thought, miracles happen.

The day before his surgery, Ted went to Mass at his parish church, Saint James in McDonough, Georgia, to pray for that miracle. He received the last rites of the church—communion, confession, and the anointing of the sick.

Ted's surgery took place on Ash Wednesday, the day in the Catholic calendar when the priest places ashes on the foreheads of the faithful and tells them, "You are dust and to dust you shall return." He arrived at the hospital at 6:00 a.m., and changed into his surgical gown.

He felt completely at peace.

Dr. Glass checked the stem cells, which had arrived by FedEx that morning. At least 80 percent had to have survived for the surgery to go forward. The results were good. There were enough living cells to proceed.

He came into Ted's room.

"Are you ready?" he asked.

"Yeah, let's do it!' Ted replied.

"Is he always this calm?" Dr. Glass asked Michelle.

Ted hugged his wife and said what could very well have been his last words to her: "Hey, I'm in love with you. I have always been in love with you. You're my best friend."

The words seemed so final, so he quickly added: "I'll see you in six hours."

With that, the nurses rolled Ted down the hallway to the surgical suite. His neurosurgeon, Dr. Nick Boulis, carefully opened a two-centimeter section of Ted's lumbar region—the lower spinal cord—while Dr. Glass drew the stem cells into a flexible tube specially designed to insert them without damaging spinal nerves.

The first injection went exactly as planned. They moved on to the second. Then the third, until one million cells had been implanted in Ted's spinal cord. Then they closed Ted up, sent him to recovery, and came out to tell Michelle the good news.

The surgery had gone exactly as planned.

Two weeks later, Ted was back at home recuperating, sitting in his favorite green recliner, when he noticed something. Before the surgery, his left leg had a deadness, a heaviness to it. But now, suddenly, the deadness, the heaviness, was missing.

"Maybe it's just because of the medication," he thought.

So he called Michelle over and asked her to push on his leg to see if he could break her strength.

This was not Michelle's favorite thing to do. Before the surgery Ted would have Michelle test his strength at home so he could see how far the disease was progressing. Each time, Ted's resistance had gotten weaker until, eventually, he could not resist even the slightest pressure from Michelle. It broke her heart to watch his decline.

Michelle sighed, and put her hand on his leg.

Ted lifted his leg with ease.

They looked at each other in disbelief.

"Maybe I didn't try hard enough," Michelle said.

Before the surgery, she never had to try at all. She would put a few fingers on his leg and was able push it down without any effort at all.

"Press harder," Ted told her.

She did.

He lifted his leg.

"Use both hands this time," Ted said.

She pressed down hard with both hands.

He lifted his leg.

The debilitating weakness was gone.

Tears started streaming down Michelle's cheeks.

"That's not supposed to happen!" she said, sobbing.

She kept saying it over and over again. "That's not supposed to happen . . . That's not supposed to happen . . . That's not supposed to happen."

"I know," Ted told her. "But it did!"

Now they were both crying.

Ted had seen joy in Michelle's eyes before—the day they were married, the day each of their kids was born. Now he saw that same joy in her eyes again.

Ted picked up the phone and called Emory. He reached Crystal, one of the clinical research coordinators.

"Crystal, tell me the truth—is anyone getting better?" he asked.

"Not that we can measure," she told him.

"Well, I am getting better," Ted told her.

Crystal told him that the surgery was a very intense procedure, and that often the more intense the procedure, the more intense the placebo effect is.

"Crystal, hear me out here. You know me. I'm not crazy. I'm a pretty rational guy. I know what a placebo effect is. This is not placebo effect."

She laughed, and told him that he was scheduled for a follow-up next week and that they would test him then. "In the meantime, whatever you are experiencing—just enjoy it while it lasts. See you Monday!"

"She thinks I'm crazy," Ted thought as he hung up the phone.

Ted went to bed that night worried that he would wake up the next day and whatever he was feeling would suddenly be gone. So every morning, Ted had Michelle test him. Not only was the feeling not gone but he kept getting stronger with each passing day.

When he arrived at Emory for his postsurgical exam, the nurses told him that since he was so insistent that he was getting better, they would go ahead and do some tests that weren't scheduled to be done yet—just to see.

"Okay! Good!" Ted said.

He smiled sportively at Michelle.

The first test they did was the hand dynamometer—to test his grip strength.

To Ted's chagrin, there was no change in his hand strength from before the surgery.

They checked his arms as well. There was no change to his upper body at all.

Ted's heart sank a little. He didn't have a hand dynamometer at home and he and Michelle had not tested his upper body. For a moment, he began to doubt.

"Who am I kidding?" he thought. "Michelle and I aren't doctors. We probably did the tests wrong."

Then they moved to his legs. The nurse pressed down on his left leg and Ted broke her strength with ease.

She looked up at him in surprise.

"What the . . . "

She called over the other nurse to try it—with the same result.

"They were looking on at me like 'What is going on?'" Ted recalls. He started laughing. "I told you!"

At that moment, Dr. Glass walked in.

"How's the patient?" he asked.

"*Really* good," the nurses said.

"Come on, doc. You've gotta check it out. It's real!" Ted told him.

Dr. Glass smiled and went over to test Ted's leg. When Ted easily broke his strength, he stepped back and stared for a moment.

He tried again. Same result.

Dr. Glass sat down in stunned disbelief. He kept running fingers through his hair, bewilderment in his eyes, Ted recalls.

"Were you trying that all the time before the surgery?" he finally asked Ted, grasping for a logical explanation.

Ted assured him he was.

"Get me all the paperwork on Harada right now. Everything we have on him," Dr. Glass told the nurses. Dr. Glass looked over the paperwork, which showed the steep decline in Ted's strength prior to the surgery. It checked out. Ted really was regaining his strength.

"I don't know what to say, I'm speechless," Glass told him.

After he recorded the results, showing Ted's miraculous turn-around, he held the chart in his hands for a moment.

"What do I do with this?" he asked.

He was holding the first medical documentation in history that showed a patient with ALS getting better.

After pausing for a moment, he signed the paperwork.

Then he looked at Ted.

"I need you to keep this to yourself right now. Don't talk about this. Don't tell anyone else."

Ted promised.

Back at home, Ted continued to feel better with each passing day. When he came back to Emory a few weeks later for his next appointment, they did all the strength tests again.

Before the surgery, Ted's hand strength had been steadily deteriorating every month. The last test before the procedure showed, on a scale of zero to 100, that his left hand was in the mid-30s and his right hand was in the mid-50s. Two weeks earlier, while doctors had found improvement in his legs, Ted's hands were exactly the same as before the surgery.

This time, when they gave Ted the hand dynamometer, he squeezed it and . . . both his hands were at 100.

The advance of ALS in his hands had been completely reversed.

The results were so unprecedented that Dr. Glass decided to go back to the beginning, and reconfirm that Ted even had ALS. In thirty years, Dr. Glass had never had a misdiagnosis. But he wanted to make sure. So he ran all the original diagnostic tests and every test came back the same way.

Ted had ALS.

"If you don't have ALS, then what you have has never been identified in the world," Dr. Glass told him.

Ted also went back to see Dr. Williams, his original neurologist at Peachtree.

"A little birdy told me you are feeling better, so let's check," Dr. Williams told him.

He conducted all the same tests that they had done at Emory—with the same miraculous results.

Ted says he had never seen a doctor drop so many expletives. With every muscle Dr. Williams pushed came a new F-word: "Holy f—! . . . What the f—!"

He finally stopped and gave Ted a big hug. He was just amazed.

Dr. Williams also reconfirmed Ted's original diagnosis. "He told me the same thing: 'Ted, there is no doubt you have ALS. There is not a doubt in my mind.'"

Dr. Glass started calling Ted at home to check in on him.

"I go to sleep thinking about you. I wake up thinking about you," he confessed.

Ted smiled. Under any other circumstance, that would be an awkward thing to hear from your doctor.

"I always thought if I found one person, they would give me the answers I was looking for," Dr. Glass told him. "But all you have given me is more questions."

Ted's quantum leaps of improvement lasted for about ten months. Then he started to get weaker again—though more gradually than before. He was like a train that had rolled up a hill and now had started slowly rolling back down again.

Since Ted's response to the first surgery was so unprecedented, Dr. Glass and his team decided to see how he would respond a second time. They asked Ted to be one of three of the original fifteen patients to undergo a second round of surgery.

On August 22, 2012, Ted went through the procedure again. This time doctors opened up the cervical area of his spinal cord—the upper area that controls respiration—and injected another 500,000 stem cells.

And this time, just like the first time, Ted's strength returned. The procedure was working.

A few months after the second surgery, Ted stood before participants at the ALS walk and shared his story.

"I think to myself: what would Lou Gehrig think today?" Ted told the crowd. "Because I'm going to walk today. . . . I'm going to walk two and a half miles. . . . So I apologize if it's a little clichéd, but I truly today can understand the words Lou Gehrig spoke so many years ago when he said, 'Today, I feel like the luckiest man on the face of the earth.'"

Ted credits both his doctors and his maker for his turnaround. "Saint John Paul II said faith and science go hand in hand because God is the author of them both," he says. "And there's no doubt that science made this happen, but I feel like faith had a part in it as well."

But if faith and science are helping him, there is one powerful force now standing in his way: the federal government.

In phase I of the clinical trials, Ted received just 1.5 million stem cells over the course of two surgeries. Doctors had wanted to use more cells, but the US Food and Drug Administration (FDA), which was supervising the trials, would not let them.

The agency forced doctors to cut the number of cells by three-quarters.

Moreover, following the success of the phase I trial, the FDA allowed doctors to dramatically increase the number of stem cells injected in phase II. Instead of 100,000 cells per injection, each patient received forty injections with 400,000 cells *per injection*. That's about 16 million cells in a single procedure—more than ten times as many as Ted received over the course of two surgeries.

If 1.5 million cells reversed Ted's ALS symptoms, imagine what 16 million cells might do for him.

But Ted won't find out anytime soon. He is not allowed to undergo the procedure again. He no longer qualifies for the study, because the date of his diagnosis is too distant and patients from the phase I trial cannot participate in phase II. And Ted cannot undergo the surgery outside the study, because the treatment has not yet been approved by the FDA.

Four years later, the procedure is still undergoing clinical trials.

"If I have shown twice that the surgery is safe and effective, why should I ever have to ask the FDA for permission to do it?" he asks. "Why should there ever be a risk they could say no to me? If I have a doctor and a drug company willing to provide this to me, and I obviously have informed consent, why should I ever be in a position where I have to go hat in hand to the FDA asking for their permission for something that has been shown to work for me twice? Why should my life rest in their hands?"

Those are good questions. And here is another.

Ted Harada is one of just thirty-two Americans who have been allowed to try this cutting-edge therapy. Many of the others have also responded well to the treatment, which has either slowed the progression of the disease or allowed them to maintain, for several years, the same level of functionality they had before the surgery.

But in the four years since the clinical trial began, twenty-four thousand people in the United States have died from ALS.

*Twenty-four thousand.*

"Every ninety minutes someone is diagnosed with ALS," Ted says, "and every ninety minutes someone dies from ALS."

The total number of Americans with ALS never changes, despite the fact that there are five thousand to seven thousand new diagnoses each year—because they all die. No one ever recovers from ALS.

But Ted Harada did recover.

So why should only thirty-two Americans with ALS have a chance to try to save their lives? How many other fathers like Ted Harada are there out there? And what about the millions of Americans with other terminal illnesses? Why are so many people dying when promising treatments exist?

What about *their* right to try?

When Ted Harada was preparing to take his miraculous two-and-a-half mile "Walk to Defeat ALS" in the fall of 2012, terminal illnesses were the furthest thing from my mind.

I had just adopted my first daughter out of the foster care system and had opened a second crib to foster another newborn. The organization I lead, the Goldwater Institute, was busy spearheading a campaign called "Save Our Secret Ballot" (S.O.S.)—passing amendments to state constitutions across the country to protect the right of workers to vote by secret ballot in elections determining if a union will represent their workforce. In Washington, federal legislation—the Secret Ballot Protection Act—was stalled on Capitol Hill. If the federal government would not do its job and protect the right to a secret ballot, we decided, states had both the authority and the responsibility to step in and do it themselves. And today, the constitutional amendment the Goldwater Institute developed has been adopted in eight states—and we have successfully defended it in federal court.

Unbeknownst to me, this success had caught the attention of a group of oncologists from Cancer Treatment Centers of America (CTCA), one of the nation's leading networks of cancer-treatment hospitals and outpatient clinics. In September 2012 they called the Goldwater Institute and said they wanted to meet with us to discuss what they said was a national medical emergency.

Then-CEO Steve Bonner told us the story of how CTCA got started.

"We were founded and are still owned by a guy named Richard Stephenson," Bonner explained. "He's an Indiana-born and -bred kid who then came to Northwestern, got a law degree, and started merchant banking, and had no real interest in health care."

But then something happened that would change the course of Stephenson's life—and the course of cancer treatment for tens of thousands of Americans. His mother, Mary Brown Stephenson, came down with a very serious form of bladder cancer. She tried all the known and approved therapies at the time, but none of them worked. So Stephenson began searching for alternative treatments.

"He was drawn to try to be helpful as a son would and looked all over the world for therapies that might be helpful to her," Bonner said. "He found a number of promising things around the world and brought them back to her bedside—and was blocked there by the FDA and by the AMA and by the insurance companies. And she died never having had a chance to avail herself of innovative therapies."

Richard Stephenson's mother was denied the right to try to save her own life.

The therapies, Bonner says, "may not have helped her but why shouldn't she have had an opportunity to try some of these things?"

The experience inspired Stephenson to found CTCA. "He wanted to create an organization that is focused truly on the patient and that everything flows from that," Bonner explained.

Now, decades later, cancer patients still face the same dilemma that Mary Brown Stephenson faced. They are being denied access to innovative treatments that could potentially save their lives. It turns out there are currently more than twenty thousand FDA trials for cancer medicines and treatments in phase II and phase III—which means they have all passed basic safety tests and many had shown efficacy in patients. But unless the drugs are already approved for another indication, it is unlawful for oncologists to use those medicines and treatments outside of those carefully controlled clinical trials, because they are not yet fully FDA approved.

Today, about 40 percent of cancer patients attempt to enroll in clinical trials, but only about 3 percent end up participating. That means the vast majority do not make the cut, whether because they fail to meet the strict criteria or a trial is thousands of miles from their home. Many of those denied access are the sickest patients—often precisely because they are too sick to be useful for study.

Worse still, the FDA takes as long as fifteen years to bring a new medicine to market. Americans are now waiting 60 percent longer for the FDA to approve life-saving medical devices—such as stents and valves—than we did ten years ago.[1]

The FDA does have a "compassionate use" policy, which is supposed to provide access to investigational treatments for terminal patients on a case-by-case basis, and the FDA believes the system works. In a 2014 radio interview, then–FDA commissioner Dr. Margaret Hamburg said, "At the FDA we are very, very concerned about patients that are suffering and their lives are at stake from devastating diseases for which they may not have an approved therapy as an option. And they have a very real need to turn to experimental treatment options. We have a long history of supporting access to experimental treatments for patients under those conditions. And we have a very good track record of approving or allowing requests for compassionate or expanded access to proceed. . . . In these instances where an individual does not qualify for a clinical trial, where there is no approved drug as a treatment for their disease and when they may need to turn to an experimental treatment option outside of the clinical trial mechanism.

"I actually do not believe that we are the barrier in these instances. . . . In fact, in many cases I actually think that FDA engagement, working with the families, working with the patient's physician, and working with the companies, have helped make expanded access actually available."[2]

No doubt FDA officials are concerned about the suffering of these patients. Like Dr. Hamburg, many of them are physicians who have dedicated their careers to curing diseases and saving lives. Their hearts are in the right place. But as we will see in the pages ahead, the system is broken.

In 2012, the year CTCA came to the Goldwater Institute, there were just 940 requests for experimental drugs approved in the entire country under the FDA's compassionate use program.[3] According to the American Cancer Society, that same year about 1,638,910 Americans were diagnosed with and about 577,190 died from cancer alone.[4] Millions more are diagnosed each year with other terminal diseases. Clearly, the system is failing to help the vast majority of Americans who are fighting to save their lives.

The FDA is a federal agency, so fixing this problem should be Congress's responsibility. But gridlock in Washington is blocking a solution. Since 2008 multiple bills have been introduced in Congress with bipartisan support to expand access for terminal patients to drugs stuck in the FDA pipeline, but most have gone nowhere.

Seeing the inaction on Capitol Hill, CTCA had come to us for help. They wanted to know if there was anything the states could do to help those dying from terminal diseases to get access to innovative treatments that could save their lives.

Bonner recalls, "I just asked the question: I wonder if there's any way to empower patients using the state authority and to give them access to care that they're otherwise not going to have access to, where they're dealing with truly a life-threatening form of the disease. If you have to go through double-blinded studies at the FDA, you know you're talking about years and people with late-stage cancer don't have years. So is there a possible exception we could carve out here for cancer patients or [others] at late stage disease?"

As I listened to Bonner and his colleagues, I immediately thought of my uncle Kenny. He died when I was about four years old from Hodgkin's lymphoma—a form of cancer for which there are now multiple treatments with very high cure rates. He was my father's only brother, and I distinctly remember my dad saying, when I was growing up, that Uncle Kenny had died just months before a new treatment was approved. At that moment it hit me: if Kenny had been allowed to try that treatment earlier, my father might still have his brother, and my cousins might still have their father.

The idea that the federal government was standing in the way of people fighting for their lives was infuriating. It's one thing for people to die because science has not come up with a treatment for their illness yet. It's quite another for someone to die when a promising treatment *exists*, but a patient can't get access to it because of governmental obstacles.

And if Washington would not fix the problem, then it was our job to step in.

The US Constitution provides a floor for freedom, not a ceiling. We can use state constitutions and powers reserved to the states to defend and expand our freedoms far above the federal baseline.

While the US Constitution protects the rights to free speech, religious liberty, and private property, many states expressly protect those freedoms to a stronger degree. Nearly every state constitution protects free speech more robustly than federal courts do under the First Amendment, protecting more types of speech and imposing a stronger burden on government to justify its censorship.

In *Federalist* number 51, James Madison wrote that a system of competing federal and state governments, each with explicit protections of individual liberties, would provide a "double security" for the rights of the people. In *Federalist* number 28, Alexander Hamilton declared, "If [the people's] rights are invaded by either [government], they can make use of the other as the instrument of redress."

The Founders understood that the rival of power is power, and the only power sufficient to rival Washington is the collective body of our fifty states. That is why they and their successors didn't give us just one Constitution—they gave us fifty-one.

I am a Goldwater conservative and a firm believer in federalism, the constitutional authority and responsibility of the states to check and balance Washington's overreach. In recent years, activists on the left have gone to the states to pass initiatives on everything from medical-marijuana legalization to the right to assisted suicide. If states have the authority to give their citizens access to marijuana and drugs to end their lives, certainly they have the authority to allow cancer patients access to investigational medicines to save their lives.

If you have the Right to Die, you have the Right to Try. And you don't have to wait for Washington to secure it.

We enthusiastically agreed to take on the project. In the months that followed, we came up with a proposal that would expand access to investigational medicines and prevail in court if challenged.

I met Dick Stephenson over lunch and explained our plan of action. Our draft law would protect a person's fundamental right to try to save his own life by expanding access to promising new drugs that await the FDA's green light if:

- the patient has a terminal diagnosis and has exhausted all conventional treatment options;
- the patient's doctor has advised that the use of an investigational treatment is the best medical option to extend or save the patient's life;
- the treatment has successfully completed basic safety testing and is part of the FDA's ongoing evaluation and approval process;
- the patient has provided "informed consent" acknowledging the potential risks associated with the use of the drug; and
- the company developing the medication is willing to make it available to the patient.

We assembled an unprecedented coalition of conservatives, liberals, and everyone in between to fight for the lives of terminal patients. And in the months that followed, Right to Try legislation has passed with overwhelming bipartisan majorities almost everywhere it has been brought up.

We knew from the beginning that Right to Try laws would be popular, but the speed with which they have taken off has been eye-opening.

When I began writing this book in the fall of 2014, Right to Try laws had been approved in five states—Colorado, Missouri, Louisiana, Michigan, and Arizona. Today, as we go to press, the number has grown to twenty-four. In those state legislatures, there have collectively been 3,045 votes in favor of Right to Try and just 26 votes against. To put that in perspective, if those were the vote totals in an election, Right to Try would have won by a margin of 99 to 1 percent.

The only place in the world you'll find results more lopsided than that is in North Korea.[5]

In Colorado, Missouri, Louisiana, Arkansas, Indiana, Mississippi, Oklahoma, Virginia, Tennessee, Texas, Nevada, North Carolina, Oregon, and Alabama, Right to Try passed without *a single dissenting vote* in either house. In Arizona, where the legislature referred it to the voters as a ballot initiative, it got 1,111,850 votes and was approved by an overwhelming 78.5 to 21.5 percent margin.[6]

Fatal diseases do not distinguish between Republicans and Democrats. Right to Try has been signed into law by both Democratic governors (Colorado's John Hickenlooper, Missouri's Jay Nixon, Montana's Steve Bullock, Minnesota's Mark Dayton, Oregon's Kate Brown, and Virginia's Terry McAuliffe) and Republican governors (Arkansas's Asa Hutchinson, Illinois's Bruce Rauner, Indiana's Mike Pence, Michigan's Rick Snyder, Louisiana's Bobby Jindal, Mississippi's Phil Bryant, Oklahoma's Mary Fallin, South Dakota's Dennis Daugaard, Utah's Gary Herbert, Wyoming's Matt Mead, North Carolina's Pat McCrory, North Dakota's Jack Dalrymple, Tennesee's Bill Haslam, Nevada's Brian Sandoval, Alabama's Robert Bentley, Florida's Rick Scott, and Texas's Greg Abbott).

We anticipate that by the end of 2015 about half the states in the Union will have Right to Try laws on the books—and the other half is soon to follow.

This book tells the story of how this movement to save lives took off, and how a relatively small grassroots organization is uniting people across the political spectrum in a fight for human dignity. In the pages that follow, we will meet courageous Americans who beat illnesses no one thought could be defeated. We will meet moms and dads who won the fight to get their children access to cutting-edge cures and those who were denied life-saving treatments by their own government. Sometimes these miracles and tragedies have taken place within the same the family.

We will meet incredible healers—doctors and medical researchers who are pioneering revolutionary cures and treatments for diseases that were once thought incurable. We will go inside the federal bureaucracy that is stopping millions of our fellow citizens from getting access to those lifesaving treatments. And we will meet some of the courageous leaders in states across this country who are fighting to give their fellow Americans the chance to save their lives.

This book is a story of medical miracles, but it is also a story of political miracles. Our country's politicians often seem to enjoy fighting and finger pointing more than problem solving. Yet in the midst of this age of pettiness and division, the Right to Try movement has united Americans of all political persuasions, and has shown that our country can still put politics aside to serve the common good.

It seems we cannot agree on much these days. But when it comes to fighting terminal illness, we can still agree on this much:

Everyone deserves the Right to Try.

# 1.

## Sophie's Choice

*How the FDA Let a Mother Save One Son . . .
and Left Her Other Son to Die*

————

Imagine the joy of watching your dying son experience a miraculous recovery thanks to an experimental medicine.

Then imagine the horror of watching your other son slowly die from the exact same disease—because the federal government prevented him from receiving the same life-saving treatment as his brother.

That is the nightmare that my friend Jenn McNary has lived for the past three years.

Jenn was a senior in high school when she had her first child, Austin. Three years later, Max came along. Jenn was a single mom, living in Vermont, struggling to support her family. She ran a child-care facility during the day and was studying child development at night school. Life was hard, but she and her young family were getting by. Both her boys seemed to be typical, healthy, happy kids.

Then, one day, Jenn began to notice that Austin was not keeping up with his friends.

"I was learning about all these age-appropriate developmental skills," she says, "like picking up a ball, standing on one foot, the ability to alternate legs going up stairs."

Austin was not meeting the developmental marks.

In the day care she ran, when all the other kids were going to the park, Austin was the only one who cried and refused to walk. He began to stumble and fall a lot and seemed to get concussions on a monthly basis. In his first-birthday picture, Jenn recalls, he had a huge bruise on his head from falling into a wall. By the age of three he had broken his arm from falling.

Jenn also noticed that Austin didn't seem to get up from the floor like the other kids. He would lift up his hips with his hands on the floor and then use his hands to crawl up his legs until he got to a standing position. He had unusually thick, muscular calves. And he crawled up stairs instead of walking like most kids his age.

Something was wrong.

It took her eight months to convince Austin's pediatrician that there was a problem, but finally the doctor agreed to have Austin tested.

One day, while Jenn was at work, the doctor called her and asked her to come in to the office. Jenn had a day care full of kids and could not get away.

"Can't you just tell me?" she said.

So the doctor told her over the phone that Austin had Duchenne muscular dystrophy.

"I don't even know what that is," Jenn said. "Is that like the Jerry's Kids thing?"

"Exactly," the doctor said.

She explained to Jenn that Duchenne was a disorder that leads to muscle degeneration and eventually death. It turned out Austin's bulging calves were not muscular at all. The muscle was breaking down and being replaced by calcium deposits that made his legs thick and hard. She explained to Jenn that there are actually forty-three different types of muscular dystrophy. Some affect children, but the majority of them affect adults. There are only a handful that are fatal.

Austin had one of the fatal ones.

Jenn asked the doctor what the treatment plan for Austin would be. "Does he need chemotherapy or something? Will he lose his hair?"

"There is no treatment," the doctor told her flatly.

Jenn was bewildered. After a long pause, she asked, "So what do I need to do?"

"You really don't need to do anything," the doctor told her. "There are no options. The disease is progressive and fatal 100 percent of the time."

Jenn was incredulous. There had to be *something* she could do. This was America, after all. Certainly in this day and age, we have treatments for everything.

She took Austin to a specialist to get a second opinion. He told her the same thing as her pediatrician. There was no treatment, no cure.

"Frankly, it's a shame you know this young," he said. "There is no benefit to you knowing this early."

"Do we need to do any more testing?" Jenn asked.

"No," the doctor told her.

"What about steroids? I read about steroid use."

The doctor got angry with her.

"Why do you want to do that to your kid? It only prolongs the inevitable."

The *inevitable*. The word hung in the air.

"So *what* do I do?" Jenn demanded. She wasn't just going to sit back and watch her son die.

"Well," the doctor told her, "when Austin is losing the ability to walk, come back and we will get him a wheelchair ordered, okay?"

Jenn couldn't believe it. She was supposed to do nothing and pretend she didn't know Austin was sick until her son lost the ability to walk? That was the plan?

"No, not okay," Jenn told him, as she stormed out of the doctor's office.

Jenn immediately began researching Austin's disease. She had no Internet access at home, so she went to the public library and started reading everything on Duchenne she could find. When she discovered that the disease was genetic, Jenn had her three-month-old, Max, tested—and found out, to her horror, that he also had Duchenne.

"I had this newborn baby who was going to die," she recalls. "I was the mother of two dying children."

Jenn became active in the Duchenne community, connecting with doctors, researchers, and other parents at conferences and online forums. And as her boys grew, and the disease progressed, she kept looking for a cure. She told herself, "By the time they are two and five years old there will be a cure." When there wasn't a cure then, she told herself, "By the time they are five and eight years old, there will be a cure." But by the time Austin turned nine and a half, she says, "I stopped thinking there was going to be a cure." Jenn pulled out of Duchenne advocacy and decided to just love her children while she still had them.

Austin began declining rapidly. But then, just as Austin turned ten years old, hope appeared on the horizon. Jenn heard about a new type of investigational therapy that appeared to be working overseas. There were two companies in London working on something called exon skipping—a treatment that coaxes cells to "skip" over the faulty sections of genetic code that causes Duchenne.

The underlying cause of Duchenne is an error in the gene that produces a protein called dystrophin that is needed to support muscle strength. Without dystrophin, ordinary physical exertion leads to muscle breakdown. As muscle fiber degenerates, children lose their ability to move—and eventually they lose the ability to breathe.

Both Austin and Max were unable to produce this critical protein, because they were missing a section of the dystrophin gene called exon 51.

Scientists in Europe were conducting clinical trials on a therapy for Austin's and Max's specific gene mutation, which affects about 13 percent of Duchenne sufferers. The scientists believed they had found a way to coax cells to skip the broken section of the gene that Austin and Max were missing. If they could do that, they might be able to restore the gene's ability to produce the vital protein.

How does exon skipping work? To understand this better, think of the genetic code for a protein as a sentence. According to Margaret Wahl of the Muscular Dystrophy Association, "Cells have to read the genetic 'sentence' in units of three 'letters' each" in order to produce the protein.[1]

The gene sentence in healthy kids would read like this:

*The mad cat ate the fat rat and the big hat.*

But kids with Duchenne have a deletion which messes up the three-letter sequence (known as the reading frame) and makes the sentence unreadable. These are called "nonsense mutations" because they turn the sentence into nonsense and make the genetic code incomprehensible.

For example, imagine that in Austin and Max the letters *fa* in "fat rat" are missing. That makes the sentence look as follows:

*The mad cat ate the tra tan dth ebi gha t.*

The cells can't read the sentence beyond the error point. And if they can't read the sentence, they can't get the instructions they need in order to produce the protein.

In exon skipping, scientists had found a way to convince the cells to skip the broken exon, or sentence fragment:

*The mad cat ate the [tra tan dth e] big hat.*

which restores the "reading frame" and produces a shorter but readable sentence:

*The mad cat ate the big hat.*

The gene is still mutated, but now the shorter readable sentence can produce a shorter but still functional dystrophin protein again.

If this new drug worked, it would transform Austin's and Max's deadly Duchenne muscular dystrophy into a much milder form of muscular dystrophy called Becker's. Their condition would become chronic instead of fatal.

Exon skipping was just the ray of hope Jenn had been looking for. As soon as she heard about it, she hopped on a plane and flew to London, where the CEOs of the two companies that were developing the exon-skipping drug were scheduled to attend a Duchenne conference.

She found them in a corner chatting and went right up to them.

"I said, 'All right, guys, my kids need this drug, which of you is going to be in the US first?'"

The two men told Jenn that they would probably be in North America about the same time, but she'd need to go to Canada to get the drug.

"I said, 'Okay, Canada it is.' And I made sure I sent both companies my kids' genetic reports."

While she was in London, Jenn also began talking to some of the parents who were participating in the clinical trial.

"All the results were great," she says. "The parents were very happy."

But one mom told her a tragic story: Her son had broken his back during the trial for one of the drugs. Because he could not walk, he was disqualified. Researchers measured how well the drug was working by comparing the patients' ability to walk before and after receiving it. That meant only kids who were ambulatory could participate in the trial.

"She was devastated," Jenn recalls, "because she was certain that the drug would have done something for her son."

Jenn's heart broke for the mom, but the news also terrified her. Austin was still ambulatory, but just barely. If he lost his ability to walk, he would not qualify for the study—just like the boy with the broken back. His window to enter a clinical trial was quickly closing.

Then, suddenly, the window slammed shut. Corporate politics and a patent fight brought the London clinical trial to a halt.[2] Jenn flew home knowing she would not get access to the promising drug she believed would save her boys. She was devastated.

"Years went by, and I really sort of lost hope again," Jenn says. "I went gray."

Within two years, Austin, then twelve, lost his ability to walk. He was now confined to a motorized wheelchair. The process of watching him lose his mobility was absolutely heartbreaking for Jenn.

"At the end stages of walking, they take maybe two or three steps and then the crumple and fall to the ground," she says. "And there is this really echoing thud that shakes the whole house, because it is dead weight. They walk and then they are on the floor. And they can't at that point get back up. So they fall to the floor and they are stuck there. And you go and lift them up."

When Austin finally decided it was time to get his power chair, Jenn says, "It was sort of a relief. He gained a lot of speed! When you aren't able to walk, and then you get this power chair that goes five miles an hour, it is pretty enlightening and freeing."

Meanwhile her other son, Max, was now nine years old. He was declining and starting to use a wheelchair occasionally as well. Jenn could see that he would soon lose his mobility, just like his older brother. It was only a matter of time. His window to a cure was closing too.

Then something happened that would change their lives.

One day in 2011 Jenn was on her computer checking Facebook when she saw a message from a friend in the Duchenne online community named Mindy Leffler. Mindy's son Aidan had been diagnosed with Duchenne in 2006 after he broke his leg playing on a slide.[3] He had the same missing exon as Max and Austin.

Mindy posted on Facebook that she was flying Aidan from their home in Bellevue, Washington, to Nationwide Children's Hospital in Columbus, Ohio.

"Fingers crossed!" Mindy wrote.

Jenn messaged her:

"Fingers crossed for what?"

Mindy wrote back that she was taking Aidan to be tested for admission into a clinical trial for an investigational drug called eteplirsen that was being developed by Sarepta Therapeutics. It was the same exon-skipping technology that Jenn learned about a few years earlier in London, targeting the precise genetic abnormality that Max and Austin suffered from.

The drug had finally made it to America!

But there was a catch. Just like in London, only ambulatory, or walking, patients qualified for the trial.

That meant it was too late for Austin. Only Max had a shot at getting in.

Jenn was determined to get the drug for Max before he lost his ability to walk. "I looked up all my old contacts and started calling," Jenn says. She began lobbying the hospital furiously, asking them to take a look at Max. She was told "no" over and over again. But she refused to take "no" for an answer. She knew this could be Max's only chance.

"I was harassing them," she says now, looking back. "And they actually said, 'Jenn, you are harassing us. We aren't even enrolling yet. We are just looking at kids.' And I said, great, I want you to look at Max." But they would not look at him.

One day she reached the principal investigator for the trial, Dr. Jerry Mendell. "What do I have to do to get you to look at Max? He's perfect. You need him," she said.

Her persistence finally paid off. "I guess you can bring him here and we will take a look at him," Dr. Mendell told her.

It was the first ray of hope she had since the London trials were canceled.

Jenn immediately got on a plane with Max and her newborn daughter (Jenn now has two other children, both of whom are healthy) and flew to the hospital in Ohio, where Max was examined. He took a test that measured how far he could walk for six minutes. If Max could not walk far enough, he would not be admitted into the trial. If he walked too far, he would also not be admitted into the trial. The investigators were looking for patients who would naturally stop walking during the course of the study—so they could see if they the drug slowed, stopped, or even reversed the progression of the disease.

Soon after returning home, Jenn got a phone call. Max had failed the walk test. He had walked too far to qualify for the trial. It was a terrible irony: to qualify, he would need to deteriorate further, but by then, it would be too late.

Max would not get the drug.

Jenn cried for two days straight. This had been Max's only hope. The rejection was as good as a death sentence.

Then, a month after being rejected, Jenn got another call from the hospital. Two participants had been disqualified, and Max could retest. This time, Max passed.

Max became patient twelve of twelve, the last child admitted into the trial.

It broke Jenn's heart that Max had to get in this way, and she vowed to herself that if this drug worked for Max, she would make it her mission to fight to get eteplirsen to everyone who needed it.

But first, she had to save her son.

Jenn began flying to Columbus from her home in Vermont once a week so that Max could receive infusions of the new drug. She used a wheelchair for Max during the trip, even though he was still walking. She was not going to let him fall and break something and get kicked out of the trial like the boy in London.

Jenn was quite a sight walking through the airport. "I have a newborn strapped to the front of me, a car seat strapped to the back of me, pushing a wheelchair and pulling a suitcase," Jenn says. "Every Tuesday morning we left. Every Wednesday he had an infusion. Every

Thursday we flew back to Connecticut and then drove to Vermont. That was our week for about a year and a half."

Max was enrolled in what is called a "double-blind placebo controlled trial," which meant that some kids in the trial were getting the drug while others were not, so that doctors could compare the outcomes. "I didn't know if he was on the drugs, on high dose, low dose, or nothing," Jenn says. She could very well have been making the arduous weekly hike from Vermont every week for an infusion of useless saline solution.

But about sixteen weeks after the infusions began, Jenn started noticing changes in Max. "The kid stopped wanting to use his wheelchair," she says. A few weeks later, he was asking to play outside—something he had not done in years. Then Max started regaining his fine motor skills. He was able to open containers again—a skill he had lost as his disease had progressed.

After about a year, he abandoned the wheelchair completely and hasn't used it since.

"Last summer he played soccer with his school soccer team," Jenn says. "This summer he is learning how to pedal a bicycle. He is able to go to the fair and walk all day long. He is able to walk through the airport. We no longer use handicap access because he just doesn't need it."

Max was getting better.

But Jenn's joy at seeing Max recover was bittersweet. At the very same time she was watching one beloved son recover, she was watching as her other beloved son continued to deteriorate.

"Austin is no longer able to transfer himself," Jenn says, her voice choking back tears. "That was something he could do [when Max joined the trial]—get into his own bed, open doors, pick things up. He was nonambulatory, but he was a really independent nonambulatory kid. He was able to dress himself in his wheelchair, roll over on his own, pull up his own blankets."

Now, at age sixteen, he could do none of those things. Every day, every week, every month that went by without the drug, Austin was losing ground.

"Pretty soon he will lose the ability to feed himself," Jenn says.

Yet amid this tragedy, something beautiful happened. As Max improved while Austin declined, the younger brother became the older one's caregiver. The boys shared a room, and Max would wake up in the middle of the night to reposition Austin in his bed or get him water. He would help Austin dress, pack his backpack, and get ready for school. If Austin needed to go to the bathroom, Max would help him transfer from his wheelchair to the toilet.

Austin didn't get the drug, but he got a brother who could help take care of him.

It has been heartbreaking for Jenn to see one of her sons improve while the other declines with each passing day. It has been even more difficult for the boys.

"Austin is very angry right now," Jenn says, "because he is not on the drug and he knows the drug works. He is angry because he is not fighting against science anymore. It is not that a treatment doesn't exist. It's just that he doesn't have access."

Jenn says Austin "doesn't understand why the grown-ups in his world can't figure this out and make things happen faster for him."

Jenn can't understand it either.

"It is one thing if your child is dying from an untreatable disease, but to have your child dying from a treatable disease is freaking devastating," she says. "I never thought it would be the government I would be working against."

Jenn worries about her family, and how Max will take it if he survives but Austin doesn't. "How is that going to affect Max?" Jenn asks. "I mean, the guilt. There was only enough drug for twelve kids; there was not enough for thirteen.

"Having a child that is dying is the most painful thing in the world. The only thing that is more painful is having a child that is dying and having a drug that could help him, and not being able to have access to it. It's a crime."

Jenn looks at her boys and sighs.

"I could have the first child in history to survive Duchenne and the last child to die from it, living in the same house."

By the summer of 2012 Jenn had had enough of watching one son get better while the other slowly declined. She decided she was going to get the drug for Austin.

And she was going to do it the only way she knew how—by cornering the CEO of the drug company.

She found out that the chief executive of Sarepta, Chris Garabedian, would be attending the annual conference of the Parent Project for Muscular Dystrophy in June 2012 in Fort Lauderdale. So she booked a plane ticket for Florida.

Garabedian was a different kind of CEO from those she had met in London. He had come to tiny Sarepta (then called AVI Biopharma) from two giants of the biotech field: Gilead Sciences and Celgene. Gilead was a pioneer in the field of antiviral medicine, developing some of the most widely used anti-AIDS drugs, and Celgene was one of the leading developers of drug therapies for cancer. The two companies were like the Apple and Google of biotech. Landing one of their top managers as CEO was a major coup for the small, struggling company.

By the time Garabedian took over in 2011, the firm was in trouble. It had spent thirty years and $250 million on research and development and didn't have a drug anywhere near FDA approval.[4] Moreover, the firm had alienated the Duchenne community. Upon his arrival, Garabedian made it his first priority to get to know the community and explain to them that the company was headed in a new direction. He was going to move forward in a very progressive, accelerated way and do everything in his power to get the drug to their children as fast as possible.

But when he arrived in Fort Lauderdale in June 2012, his prospects for doing so looked dim. Sarepta was struggling to stay afloat. The company's stock was down 30 percent. He was running out of cash. Garabedian couldn't find any investors to give him the money he needed to keep Sarepta in the black.

He didn't know if Sarepta was going to survive.

Worse, he didn't know if he even had a product. Eteplirsen had completed a phase I trial, which proved that the drug was safe. But the clinical signal—the actual improvement in function of the patients—from that initial trial was not strong. Garabedian was betting everything he had on the tiny, twelve-patient phase II trial that Max was in.

Even putting that trial together had been a struggle. When he first took over the company, Garabedian told the BioBeat blog, he had called up his head of manufacturing and asked how much of the drug they had in stock.

"Not much," the department head told him.

"How much is not much?" Garabedian asked.

"We have enough to treat eight patients for about twenty-four weeks," he said.

That was not good.

"How long will it take to get more drug?" Garabedian asked nervously.

"Nine months to a year," came the reply.[5]

With a limited supply of drug and no capacity to make more quickly, Garabedian took what he had and came up with the best small trial he could design. The study would enroll twelve patients. Eight would get the drug, while four more would be placed in a placebo control group.

To put this in perspective, his nearest competitor, Prosensa and its pharmaceutical partner, GlaxoSmithKline, were conducting a 180-patient study for its drug, which was targeting a different flaw in the exons. It was just the kind of large, double-blind randomized trial the FDA favored.

A large trial like that was out of reach for Garabedian. His little twelve-patient study would have to do. If the data showed his drug worked, he could raise money to scale up production, move the four patients in the placebo group onto the drug, and keep the study going.

If not, Sarepta could be finished.

When Garabedian flew to Fort Lauderdale, it was early in the study and he had no idea if his drug was working . . . until, that is, Jenn McNary cornered him.

"I was approached by a mom I had never met or heard of at the time, Jenn McNary," Garabedian explained in an interview with *Boston Business Journal*. "She approached me in the summer of 2012, before the company even had its 36-week data that was the first signal of a clinical efficacy. And she told me, 'Your drug is working. My son is in your trial.'"

Jenn recalls the moment. "I didn't know him, but I waved him over. I said, 'You're the CEO of Sarepta, right? Great, my son is getting better and your drug works.' And he looks at me and goes, 'We don't have the data to back that up yet.' I said, 'Oh, I have the data. He lives with me. It works.'"

Jenn told Garabedian how Max had gone from using a wheelchair half the time to playing in the yard with his siblings. She also told him about Austin, who did not qualify for the trial because he was already wheelchair bound, and how desperately he needed the drug.

Garabedian was moved by Austin's plight, but he explained that he literally didn't have any drug to give him. Sarepta was barely able to churn out enough to keep Max going in the trial. He didn't have any cash, didn't have any drugs, and didn't have any manufacturing capacity. The company was on its final breath. He was rolling the dice on Max's trial. They needed data showing a separation between the placebo-delayed group and the early treatment group in the trial, or there would be no more drug, period.

Garabedian later told reporters that his conversation with Jenn was the first evidence he had that his drug was working. "She saw what [the company] didn't see, and the rest of the marketplace and DMD community didn't see, because she had a boy in our study."[6]

A month after speaking with Jenn, in July 2012, Garabedian finally got some desperately needed good news. The thirty-six-week analysis of Max's trial showed the clinical signal he had been hoping for. Four boys on the highest dose of eteplirsen saw their walking ability decline by just 8.7 meters, compared with a decline of 78 meters in walking ability for boys who were not on the drug.

Eteplirsen had dramatically slowed their decline. When Sarepta announced the interim results, its stock went up 150 percent.

Then, three months later, the forty-eight-week data came out, and the news was even better. The clinical outcomes were unprecedented. Boys on the drug were able to walk an average of 21 meters *farther* than at the start of the study, and 89 meters farther than those on placebo.[7]

Moreover, muscle biopsies showed that levels of dystrophin—the protein they had been missing to repair their muscles—in the boys on the drug were increasing significantly. Two boys, a set of twins, had not been able to benefit from the treatment. But all the other boys were doing phenomenally well.

Dr. Mendell, the principal investigator, hailed the results, saying the data "represent a significant milestone and a defining moment of progress and hope for patients with DMD and their families." Eteplirsen, he said, "has demonstrated unparalleled effects on enabling dystrophin production and slowing the progression of the disease."[8]

Everyone from the placebo-delayed group was now getting the drug. The moms started tweeting, posting videos, spreading the word: Eteplirsen was working.

Jenn recalls, "The day the forty-eight-week data came out, I called him and said, 'Great, now you know it works. So what are you gonna do? I have this other kid who is still dying. You have to help.'"

But he could not help. Unlike pharmaceutical giants like GlaxoSmithKline, he did not have the money to scale up production. The only way he could raise enough cash to do so was if the FDA gave Sarepta a green light for accelerated approval of the drug. Then the stock would go up, and Garabedian could raise money in anticipation of the drug's being approved, produce the drug, and have it ready to sell immediately on approval.

As word spread on social media of eteplirsen's success, Sarepta was inundated with requests like Jenn's. So Garabedian issued an open letter to the Duchenne community explaining the company's predicament:

> We know that drug development is a painfully drawn-out process for those who are waiting and we take seriously our responsibility to act as a true partner of the DMD community as we move forward together. We are currently producing eteplirsen at a scale that is sufficient to meet the needs of the 12 patients in this study. . . . At the present time, we do not have excess drug supply to make eteplirsen available outside of a clinical trial setting on a compassionate use basis.

"We can only imagine how difficult this is to hear, but unfortunately we have no other options available to us right now," he continued. The only way to get the drug to people who needed it, Garabedian explained, was to "advance this therapy through the regulatory process and, ultimately, secure approval for all DMD patients who would benefit."[9]

When she read Garabedian's letter, Jenn was heartbroken. But she also realized Sarepta was not holding out on her. It could not afford to produce the drug on a wider scale until the company knew that there was a pathway for approval. And the only agency that could clear that pathway was the Food and Drug Administration. The FDA had the authority to get the drug to her son or withhold it. The FDA held the power of life and death. So Jenn decided that is where she would focus her energy from here on out. Instead of targeting the company, Jenn would target the FDA and focus on convincing it to accelerate the approval of eteplirsen.

Fortunately, Congress had recently passed a new law that could help her do just that. On July 9, 2012—the same month Sarepta announced its thirty-six-week findings—President Barack Obama signed the Food and Drug Administration Safety and Innovation Act (FDASIA). The law created a new designation at the FDA for "breakthrough therapies" and encouraged the agency to speed the review of new drugs for fatal diseases by measuring a "surrogate" outcome (such as how much dystrophin Duchenne boys are producing) instead of a "clinical" outcome (how far they can walk).

If a drug meets a surrogate outcome—or "end point" in the FDA's terminology—it strongly suggests that eventually the clinical outcome of improving how patients feel, function, or survive will also be met. For example, the lack of dystrophin is the cause of Duchenne. So if a drug helps Duchenne kids start producing dystrophin, it is likely that they will eventually meet the clinical outcome of walking farther. In clinical trials, the surrogate outcome is usually reached before the clinical one. You can measure how much dystrophin the body is producing long before the protein starts to have a measurable impact on muscle function—and thus progress in a six-minute walk test.

The new law encouraged the agency to approve breakthrough drugs on the basis of the surrogate outcome, so patients can get access to the drug faster. Then the agency can require additional studies after approval to confirm that the clinical outcome had been achieved as well.

Sarepta would be one of the first companies to seek accelerated approval for a breakthrough therapy under the new law. Congress had just sent clear instructions to the FDA: accelerate approval of treatments for rare diseases. Now Garabedian's company was going to ask the FDA to live up to Congress's mandate and approve eteplirsen on the surrogate goal of dystrophin production.

Garabedian knew this would not be easy. FDA officials were

ambivalent about accelerated approval to begin with. The neurological division of the FDA, which had the final say over his drug, had not granted accelerated approval to any drug since 2004. It was not clear how the division would respond to the new directive from Congress. The law had *authorized* but did not *require* accelerated approval based on surrogate markers for breakthrough drugs.

He and his company were entering uncharted territory.

"We were testing the intent of [the law]," Garabedian says, and when you're "one of the first to try to apply legislation like FDASIA, it's tough. It's tough on all parties to be the first. And you're trying to run through that wall. And you're going to get hurt. But once you crack through that wall, and allow others to follow, if it's done the right way and it's an appropriate application, it's for the benefit of all."[10]

There was another important change under the new law: Congress had created a new role for patients and disease advocacy groups.

"One of the aspects of FDASIA was to encourage the FDA to open its doors and meet more often with patients groups because the legislation wanted it to be considered as part of the drug approval process," Garabedian says.

That meant FDA officials had to meet with Jenn McNary.

So not only did Sarepta's case become the first test of a company seeking accelerated approval for a rare disease under the new law; it was also the first test of the patient community engaging the FDA since FDASIA was passed.

If Jenn was going to take on the federal government, she could not do it alone. She needed reinforcements.

And her son Max was about to help her find them.

Just before Max began his clinical trial, he and Austin had been invited to attend a special weeklong overnight camp for kids, teens, and adults with muscular dystrophy. Camp Promise was a program of the Jett Foundation, a small charity started by a Boston-area nurse named Christine McSherry and named for her son Jett.

"When I had my son he appeared perfectly normal and healthy," Christine says. "The first couple of years were very uneventful. He was growing. He had beautiful blue eyes and big eyelashes and blond hair. He was a spitting image of my husband and it was like falling in love with my husband all over again."

Christine's house was always in a state of barely controlled chaos. Jett was the third of five children, and his two little brothers were a whirlwind of hyperactivity.

"You would leave the room and come back and all the furniture would be rearranged or upside down," Christine says. "And Jett would just be sitting there like 'I don't know what happened.' So I really thought Jett was just a mellow kid and the others were not."

There were no signs of trouble. Jett walked on time, crawled on time; he could run, play sports, and ride a bike. "There was really nothing significant to set us off—other than he had trouble getting up off the floor and his calves were a little enlarged," Christine says.

When Jett turned five, Christine took him to the pediatrician's office for his annual well check. That day, she says, "my world changed."

The pediatrician became concerned watching Jett get up off the floor in his office. Just like Austin, Jett put his hands on his knees and used them to crawl up his legs to a standing position.

"Oh dear, we have a problem," the doctor told Christine.

The pediatrician sent Christine to a neurologist, who drew Jett's blood. When the results came in, Jett's CPK level was off the charts. In muscular dystrophy, the muscles in the body break down and release the CPK enzyme, which is the signal that the muscles are dying. Christine is a registered nurse, and when she saw the results, she says, "I thought immediately there must be a mistake because you can't have a CPK level that high—even in a heart attack."

Unless, that is, you have Duchenne muscular dystrophy.

She watched Jett jumping on and off the examining table as she tried to take in the crushing news: Jett was dying.

"The doctor told me there wasn't a drug or a treatment that I could give him," she says. "I was a nurse for a long time. I was very accustomed to finding the solution and giving it to the patient, and was shocked to find out that there was no solution whatsoever."

Christine was told that Jett would not be likely to make it past the age of fifteen.

That weekend, Christine and her husband told their family and friends they were going skiing. "But in fact we put the cars in the garage, we drew the blinds in the house, and we shut off all the lights, and we sat in the bed for an entire weekend, and just mourned. The kids sat in bed with us and we all ate Cheerios and watched cartoons on TV in mom and dad's bed for an entire weekend. The kids slept there and everything. We all just slept together and mourned."

When Monday arrived, Christine's husband decided to go to work. "I've got to do something productive," he told her. She told him she understood.

Later that morning, when the babysitter arrived, Christine took Jett, put him in the car and headed to Cape Cod.

"I never understood, even when I was a nurse, how much pain people were in to want to kill themselves," she says. "There were many suicide attempts that came into the hospital where I worked. I would take care of those patients, but I could never understand what could cause so much hurt to make them want to kill themselves. They would say that the pain was just too bad. How could they be in that much pain? That Monday morning I understood exactly what those patients were talking about."

She drove to the Sagamore Bridge that connects Cape Cod with the mainland of Massachusetts across the Cape Cod Canal. Christine remembered driving across the bridge as a little girl and seeing the big blue sign at either end that read "Desperate? Call the Samaritans."

"All I could think is that I just had to end my life, Jett's life, because I couldn't let the other four children go through watching their brother die. And I certainly couldn't have their father, who I love so much, witness the same thing. There must be something better."

She just sat there in the car, staring at the bridge.

Jett looked at her.

"What are we doing here, Mom?" he asked.

"I'm not really sure," Christine told him.

"Well, let's take a walk, Mom," Jett said.

So Christine parked the car and together they walked down to the causeway, sat down, and stared out at the water.

It was a cold February morning, so she and Jett were all alone. As she sat there, she imagined what it would be like for her girls to hear that mom was not coming back, that their little brother was not coming back.

"And for some reason, I just had the revelation that maybe somehow we could survive this," Christine says. "Maybe I could do something to help my family survive it even if Jett did not survive."

Perhaps, she thought, she could turn the pain she was feeling into something productive—something that could help Jett, help her family, and help others.

Christine and Jett got back into her car and came home. And slowly, her despair turned into determination.

"I wasn't going to let him die like they told me he would," Christine says. "Being able to throw a ball, being able to ride a bike, being able to walk, being able to go to the prom, being able to become a man, to have a career, have children. There had to be something that we could do."

So she started the Jett Foundation. "We picked the logo of the fighter plane because we were determined that we were going to fight this."

Over the next fifteen years, the foundation grew—and so did Jett. His disease progressed more slowly than Christine had anticipated.

"He was able to play a lot of sports," she says. "He played baseball, he played soccer, he swam, he participated on a ski team. We tried to give him everything that we thought that he could potentially do. Because eventually, you know, all you have left when they go is memories. So we wanted to create as many memories for him as possible."

As Jett got older, so did his awareness of the seriousness of his condition. One day, he was alone on the computer and decided to look up his disease. "He typed in 'Duchenne' and it said 'fatal before the age of 19,'" Christine says. "And we walked into his room, and he was throwing things around and just going crazy." Christine tried to comfort him. She told him it would be all right. She had a plan, she was working hard to save his life, it wasn't going to end that way for him.

Jett screamed at her: "What makes me so special? What makes me so special? What makes you think that that can happen?"

From that moment, Christine gave up everything in her life except fighting for Jett—no more dinners, birthday parties, baseball games, visiting her parents. "I was 125 percent in," she says. "I just gave up years and years and years of being a mommy."

Like Jenn McNary, she kept waiting for a cure that never seemed to come. "I had in my mind the entire time all these years that a treatment would happen just in the nick of time."

As Jett progressed in his disease, she watched him losing his independence. And through her work in the Jett Foundation, she saw other kids doing the same.

"As a nurse my instinct has always been to try to help other people," she says. So Christine started reaching out to local sports teams and organizing events for Duchenne kids. The Boston Bruins invited the kids on the ice in their power chairs for a skate. The New England Patriots hosted them for a special Duchenne day at the Patriots training camp.

One day, Christine noticed that the Muscular Dystrophy Association camp stopped at age seventeen—and she thought about all the Duchenne kids she knew who had beaten the odds and made it to nineteen or twenty. They didn't qualify for camp anymore. Christine decided to start a camp of her own that would be open to kids and adults of all ages. And in 2009, Camp Promise was born.

"There was this family in Vermont who I knew of through Facebook," Christine says. They would come to some of her events. And they came to the first year of Camp Promise.

Christine remembers keeping a special eye on Max that week.

"I watched him specifically because he was in that transition age where you go from being ambulatory to not ambulatory," Christine recalls. "And it can be very difficult because kids will often fall. And when kids with Duchenne fall, they spontaneously collapse. It's not like they trip over anything, or there's a sign of weakness when they fall. They just all of the sudden fall for no reason. Their legs go out from under them. It's scary as anything. A lot of kids end up breaking their bones, because they can't even brace themselves for the fall because they don't know it's coming."

The last thing she wanted was for any of the kids to fall and get seriously injured at her first camp, so she watched Max like a hawk.

"I was probably a little bit more cautious with him than most kids," she says, "so I had a very good idea of what his skill set was and what he could do and what he couldn't do."

The following year, Max did not come to Camp Promise, but he did come to Patriots Day training camp.

Christine recalls what happened next. "We gathered everybody down in the parking lot and then we started walking down toward the practice field. And as we were approaching the practice field, I noticed Max actually ran past me. I couldn't understand it. I was like, 'All right, wait a minute, is this the same kid?'"

She grabbed her phone and looked up some pictures from camp the previous year just to make certain she had the right kid.

"Sure enough it was him," she says.

Christine spent the rest of the day watching Max. "Max was doing some things that you wouldn't expect a child who had previously spent more than half their time in some sort of a mobility device to be doing. He was goofing off with his little sister and his little brother and jumping on and off a little wall and climbing on the wall."

She remembers Jenn McNary getting a little bit irritated with Max, telling him, "Would you stop it? Would you just sit down?" Christine kept thinking, "Don't make him sit down! Don't make him sit down! He's moving! This is amazing!"

She didn't say anything to Jenn, but when she got home she went back on Facebook and looked at Jenn's profile. She saw what Jenn had posted about the clinical trial Max was in, how he was getting better, and how she could not get the drug for Austin. She was reaching out to the online Duchenne community for help.

So Christine sent Jenn an email. "I told her I agree there's a change in Max and I know that because I saw him at camp last year. And I said, listen, I'll help you because I believe that Jett would also be amenable to that exon and let's team up and see what we can do together."

Jenn had been running into brick walls in the wider Duchenne community. She wanted to get *all* the Duchenne organizations behind eteplirsen. So she approached the Muscular Dystrophy Association, the Parent Project Muscular Dystrophy (at whose conference she had first met Chris Garabedian), and other leading Duchenne groups, and asked for their help in a campaign to get eteplirsen approved.

They all turned her away.

"I was told by leaders from major Duchenne organizations that I was not going to be useful. That I am undereducated. I am not a nurse. I am not anything. I never went to college," Jenn says. "I was told several times: you are just a mom of two kids, you don't belong in the halls of Congress. You don't belong on TV talking about this. You don't belong at the FDA trying to make a point. Leave that to the experts."

Christine says, "She was doing her best to reach out to every organization and they were doing their best to dissuade her. She finally just realized that these people are not doing what's best for Austin. So we started working together."

They worked remotely at first, Jenn from Vermont and Christine from Boston.

"We reached out to everyone, everywhere we could, and kind of got a master's degree in FDA relations, policy, everything that you can imagine so that we could be effective," Christine says.

Then, in the spring of 2013, Jenn's life shattered. She had gotten married after Max and Austin were born, but now her husband told her he wanted a divorce. He left her all alone with four children—two of them with a fatal illness—and no income.

Jenn called Christine in a panic. "She's like 'I can't do this. I can't do this alone. I don't have any money. I don't know what to do. I don't have a job. I can't get a job. I can't take Max to his infusion.'"

Christine knew that if Jenn could not take Max to his infusion, Max would lose all the incredible progress he had made. Worse still, the study would be compromised, and the chances of the FDA approving the drug would be set back. There were only twelve kids in the trial, so losing one—especially one in whom the drug was working—would have been catastrophic.

So Christine swung into action. "I said pack everything that you can pack and I will be there in like a week and I will move you to my town," Christine says.

Where would she live? Jenn asked. She had never lived anywhere but Vermont.

Christine told her, "I don't know. I'll figure it out. Don't worry about it. I'm going to be there with a truck in a week. You've got a week to pack up."

Christine found Jenn an apartment in her hometown and helped her get the boys signed up for school. "I knew, one, I could give her a job; two, eventually we'd get the infusions transferred down to the Boston area so it would be closer; three, she would be safe and she would have housing; and four, her kids would go into the school system where Jett had already been and they understood Duchenne. So there wasn't going to be a problem."

Jenn went to work full-time at the Jett Foundation as an advocate for Duchenne families. That gave Jenn a way to support her family and keep Max in the trial. Even more important, it also meant she was no longer just a lone single mom confronting CEOs at conferences or fighting the federal government on her own. Now she was part of a team.

Now she had reinforcements.

Suddenly, Jenn was meeting with senators and congressmen, testifying before the FDA, and meeting with its top leaders—all the things the Duchenne community had told her it was not her place to do. And Jenn blossomed in her new role.

"She found her voice," Christine says.

Jenn began to apply the same tenacity that got Max into that clinical trial to helping Austin and other Duchenne kids get the same lifesaving treatments. Her goals expanded. Not only would she get Austin the drug; she was going to make the FDA approve the drug so that every kid like Austin could get it as well.

She and Christine began recruiting more Duchenne moms into their growing campaign.

First, they brought Mindy Leffler, Jenn's Facebook friend who had told her about the Sarepta trial, into the fold. It turned out that Mindy's son, Aidan, had been rejected for the Sarepta trial—not for being too sick, but for being too *healthy*.

Jenn says, "They were choosing children that walked less than four hundred meters in a six-minute walk test because they were trying to choose children that naturally would stop walking during the course of a trial." The irony was surreal: Austin did not qualify because he could not walk at all; Aidan did not qualify because he could walk *too far*.

After Aidan was turned down, Mindy and her husband, Mitch, scrambled to join the trial for the competing drug being developed by

Prosensa.[11] For forty-eight weeks, they took Aidan back and forth between Bellevue and Vancouver, British Columbia, where the trial was being held. When he didn't have the same side effects as the other kids, Mindy figured out that Aidan was probably on the placebo—which meant she was likely going back and forth to Canada every week for an infusion of saline solution. And when all the boys in the placebo group were finally put on the drug, Mindy didn't see any meaningful progress in Aidan's condition.

Then, without warning, the study was shut down. "No one called us," Mindy told *Businessweek* at the time. "We learned the trial was over from a GSK [GlaxoSmithKline] investor conference call. . . . There's no safety net. You just crash."

Mindy realized her best hope for Aidan was to get him eteplirsen. So she teamed up with Christine and Jenn and the other Duchenne moms to fight for FDA approval. "I want Aidan on that drug and I want it to happen before he's in a wheelchair or worse," she said.[12]

The moms quickly found Tracy Seckler, whose son Charley had been diagnosed with Duchenne and who had started her own foundation—Charley's Fund—that had raised millions for Duchenne research. Then came Marissa Penrod, whose youngest son, Joseph, had been diagnosed with Duchenne. Neither Charley nor Joseph could benefit directly from eteplirsen, since both were missing a different exon from the one Austin, Max, and Jett were missing. But Tracy and Marissa knew that Sarepta's technology would work on other exons as well. Once the FDA approved eteplirsen, it would help clear the way to approval for Sarepta's follow-on therapies.

Together, this growing army of Duchenne moms launched a campaign they called the "Race to Yes" to press the FDA to approve eteplirsen.

They chose the Duchenne community's hourglass as their symbol, because time was what they were up against.

While the moms mobilized their growing forces, eteplirsen continued showing progress in clinical trials. But instead of fast-tracking the drug for speedy approval, the FDA played "Lucy with the football."

After the forty-eight-week results came out in October 2012, Jenn had launched a petition on Change.org demanding accelerated approval of the drug. By February 2013 her petition had collected more than 170,000 signatures.

A month later, Sarepta made its first formal presentation to the FDA. Chris Garabedian, Sarepta's then-CEO, said, "We could have been told, 'No chance, go back and do a large placebo-controlled study, come back and talk to us in a few years.'"[13] Instead, the response was encouraging.

On April 15, 2013, Sarepta announced, "The FDA has requested that Sarepta provide additional information from the existing Eteplirsen dataset to inform a decision on the acceptability of this dataset for a New Drug Application (NDA) filing under . . . Accelerated Approval."[14]

This announcement was good news, but it—and the ones that followed—became a source of tension between the company and the FDA. As part of his commitment to transparency with his investors and the Duchenne community, Garabedian decided to make all the company's interactions with the FDA public. Every time Sarepta executives interacted with the FDA, the company would put out a press release detailing the outcome of the meeting, including any guidance the agency gave it or data the FDA requested.

Investors appreciated the unprecedented transparency because the company's stock was tied almost exclusively to whether or not the FDA was supportive of accelerated approval. The Duchenne community appreciated the transparency because, as Christine put it, "it gave us the fuel that we needed to go back to the FDA and argue their point." When the agency would raise objections—for example, questioning whether dystrophin is important—the Duchenne moms would enlist scientists and provide data proving that dystrophin was in fact important.

The only party that didn't like the transparency was the FDA. Christine says, "The agency did not like us knowing all the communications between the company and them. They did not like the fact that the company was able to highlight some of their ignorance around personalized medicine and Duchenne in general. They did not like the fact that the advocates—we were now called 'the advocates'—knew more about the drug and about the data than they did. Because that's what we were doing 24/7. We were eating it for breakfast, basically. And the agency and the neurology division were looking at other drugs other than just eteplirsen."

As Sarepta engaged with the FDA, the Duchenne moms launched a full-court lobbying press. They held congressional briefings, organized letters from members of Congress to the FDA, and had seven conversations in six months with Dr. Janet Woodcock, the director of the FDA's Center for Drug Evaluation and Research. In fact, the moms were getting more time with the FDA hierarchy to discuss eteplirsen than the company was.

At first, their efforts seemed to pay off. On July 24, 2013, Sarepta announced that the FDA had provided the company with official guidance indicating that it would be open to a new drug application (NDA) for eteplirsen later in the year.

"We are encouraged by the feedback from the FDA and believe that data from our ongoing clinical study . . . will be sufficient for an NDA filing," Garabedian declared in a press statement.[15]

The Duchenne moms were elated. It looked like the drug was finally moving forward toward accelerated approval.

In October, both Christine McSherry and Dr. Janet Woodcock were honored at a gala hosted by the EveryLife Foundation—Christine for her advocacy and Dr. Woodcock for her work advancing faster drug-approval pathways. Jenn and Christine brought their kids to the gala. It was the first time Dr. Woodcock got to meet Max, Austin, and Jett. They posed together for pictures. Everyone was smiling. The system appeared to be working.

The smiles did not last long, however. A month after the gala, the

FDA pulled the football away. *Businessweek* reported that FDA "evaluators . . . told Sarepta not to bother applying for approval."[16] The decision was based, in part, on the failure of its competitor's clinical trial. Sarepta tried to explain how its drug was different from the competitor's and to show why the data from its studies was compelling, but the evaluators would not budge. They said that an application for accelerated approval would be "premature."[17]

The moms felt betrayed. They had been meeting with Dr. Woodcock and senior FDA officials for months and were getting nothing but encouraging signals. The setback came as a complete surprise. They felt they had been lied to.

Not ones to back down, they ramped up the pressure on the FDA. Christine recalls some of the tactics they employed.

"There was the day when Jenn published Janet Woodcock's phone number on Facebook and told everybody to call on a Monday morning at 9:00 a.m. and literally shut down the phone system at the FDA," she says. "We got an email from Janet's assistant that said, 'We got the message. Could you guys please tell people to stop calling my line?' Then there was another time when we asked everybody to email the agency and I believe we shut down their server for a couple of hours."

They also took advantage of a system President Obama had established allowing citizens to start online petitions on the White House website. Any petition that got 100,000 signatures within thirty days would get an official response from the White House. So in February the moms launched a White House petition urging the FDA to "say yes" to a cure for Duchenne.[18]

By the end of March, they had gathered 106,782 signatures, enough to force an official response.

At the same time that they launched their White House petition, the moms brought seven of the world's Duchenne experts to Washington to meet with FDA officials. They came from Perth, London, and Toronto, and included the Harvard professor who discovered dystrophin in 1987.

"If the government officials won't listen to us, we reasoned, surely they would listen to the experts," Tracy Seckler explained in an op-ed for the *Huffington Post*. "All in attendance . . . agreed that Eteplirsen is producing the missing protein. All agreed that producing dystrophin is more than 'reasonably likely' to lead to clinical benefit. All agreed that we are in fact already seeing clinical benefit in the 12 boys exposed to treatment."[19]

Once again, it seemed that the petition and the meetings had an impact. In April 2014 the FDA reversed itself and once again invited Sarepta to submit an NDA later that year.[20]

Soon after the announcement, Dr. Woodcock issued the official response to the Duchenne moms' White House petition—and, not surprisingly, she touted the FDA's decision:

> We share your sense of urgency to make safe and effective drugs available for patients with Duchenne muscular dystrophy as soon as possible. That's why we're actively engaged with a number of drug companies focused on developing new drugs for Duchenne muscular dystrophy, including Sarepta Therapeutics, the company developing eteplirsen. . . . Sarepta Therapeutics has publicly announced its intention to file a New Drug Application for eteplirsen by the end of 2014 as well as plans to initiate several additional clinical studies with eteplirsen later this year. As mentioned above, we are willing to explore the use of all potential pathways for the approval of drugs for Duchenne muscular dystrophy (including accelerated approval) as appropriate.

The moms had not even mentioned eteplirsen in their petition, yet Woodcock cited the drug by name. They were thrilled that eteplirsen was back on track for accelerated approval.

Alas, their victory was short-lived. A few months later, the FDA pulled the football back once again—withdrawing the guidance inviting an NDA and demanding even more data.

The agency told Sarepta that it could apply in mid-2015.

Christine says, "The agency was getting so upset that the company kept releasing the information about their meetings and how they kept asking for additional data, additional data, additional data that they actually became somewhat vindictive. It seemed like the more we pushed, the more things they asked for, so we backed off a little bit."

When the moms complained about the delay, they were told it was just six months.

"What does that mean?" Tracy Seckler, Charley's mom, said during a Google chat organized by the Jett Foundation following the decision.

It's not just six months, it's six *more* months added onto the delays we've already endured. [And] once the New Drug Application is filed, the review process, if it's expedited takes *another* six months. And [then] we already know it takes six months for Eteplirsen to start producing dystrophin. So from today it's going to be another year-and-a-half before all eligible children can start benefitting from Eteplirsen. That's another year-and-a-half on top of the year-and-a-half we have already spent fighting.

The only analogy I can think of that comes close to this is the *Titanic*. Our children are on the *Titanic* and we know it's going down with 100 percent certainty. There's a lifeboat and a team of engineers has reviewed the lifeboat and said it's reliable. We need to get the kids into these lifeboats instead of questioning every single bit of minutia about the way the lifeboat was developed. Because while we're asking those questions, the kids on the *Titanic* are going down. Let's work together to get more lifeboats in the water and to get every kid a chance to keep them afloat; better and stronger lifeboats will come along but what good will it do if we leave our kids on the *Titanic* while we're waiting for them?

Marissa Penrod, Joseph's mom, said, "The FDA is failing our children. Every passing second, every day, every minute, ever hour, children with Duchenne are losing muscle. My ultimate fear is that my little boy will lose the ability to hug me. He walked across the room to me over the weekend and about five feet before he got to me his legs just gave out without warning. He buckled and went to the ground."

Her message to the FDA? "Our children can no longer be your science experiment. The children are not here to serve science. The science should always serve the children."

Yet nearly three years after Sarepta first demonstrated that eteplirsen was safe and helping Duchenne kids, the FDA still had not invited Sarepta to apply for approval of the drug.

How many kids were being hurt by the FDA's delays? There are about fifteen thousand to twenty thousand boys in the United States with Duchenne, and eteplirsen can help about 13 percent of them. That is about 1,950 to 2,600 boys who desperately need this drug.

But that is only scratching the surface. Sarepta estimates that its broader portfolio of exon-skipping compounds—all based on the same technology as eteplirsen—could help about 80 percent of those boys.[21] That's twelve thousand to sixteen thousand kids in the United States alone—and tens of thousands more across the globe who could benefit.

But today, Jenn says, "There are only twelve children in the world receiving that medicine. The rest of the children are wasting away and dying."

That, she says, is unacceptable. "Kids die from this disease every day. I know at least two personally who have died [since Max's clinical trial began] who needed this drug. Five children with Duchenne died last week that I know of. Of course, there are more that we don't know personally. This is not hypothetical. This is children dying every day."

Jenn continues to fight for those kids, and her own, but the fight has taken its toll.

"This has not been an easy road," she says. "It caused a divorce in my life. It brings me away from my family. But I think that it was very important to speak up. I very, very strongly believe that if I had never said to the public, 'Hey this drug exists! It's working and we deserve access!' nobody would know about it."

While she is confident she will ultimately prevail, she is also aware that success may come too late for her son.

"This may not make a change for Austin. He may be too far gone by the time he does get on the drug," Jenn says. "But hopefully, I will save some kids who are just being diagnosed right now. And they may never have to experience the symptoms of this disease."

Unfortunately, Jenn, Christine, Mindy, Tracy, and Marissa were not alone in their struggle with the federal government. Halfway across America, in Phoenix, Arizona, an eleven-year-old boy was about to launch an epic battle to save his own life—a battle that would ultimately help him save the lives of countless others.

# Five Thousand Miles for a Cure

*How One American Family Moved Overseas*
*to Save Their Dying Son*

———

How far would you go to get a drug that could save your child's life? Halfway across the world? Unfortunately, that is exactly what the government is forcing some families with dying children to do.

Like many young kids, Diego Morris is a sports fanatic. He has a Phoenix Suns blanket on his bed and Larry Fitzgerald's Arizona Cardinals jersey on the wall of his room. A dual-sport athlete, he loved playing both soccer and Little League baseball.

One morning, when he was eleven, Diego woke up with intense pain in his left knee. At first his parents, Paulina and Jason, figured it was a sports injury. They gave him some Advil and an ice pack and waited to see if it got better.

When the pain didn't go away, they decided to take him to the pediatrician to have it checked out just in case.

"I have to tell you, it didn't faze me," says Diego's father, Jason. "Of course his knee is bothering him. He's a tough kid, he plays aggressively."

Paulina brought Diego to the doctor's office. When the pediatrician touched his knee, Diego yelped in pain. She had known Diego all his life and had never seen him respond this way. So she sent him to an orthopedic surgeon, who took an X-ray.

It wasn't a sports injury.

"The orthopedic surgeon turned to me after looking at the X-ray, and he was white as a ghost," Paulina says. "He said, 'I think this is serious.'"

Paulina gave Diego her iPad and told him to go play in the lobby while she and the doctor talked. When he left, the doctor closed the door to the examining room. He sat Paulina down and told her that, while he'd have to take an MRI to confirm it, the X-ray indicated Diego had osteosarcoma—a rare bone cancer.

Cancer? Paulina thought. A few minutes ago she was worried he might have twisted his knee on the soccer field. Now he was facing a life-threatening diagnosis.

She immediately called Jason, who was picking Diego's brother Mateo up from school, and told him to come to the doctor's office at once.

"I was driving home with Mateo when Paulina called and she was in tears and I could hear it in her voice immediately, she was scared to death," he says. He rushed over to join her.

Paulina says that the doctor "ran us down to the MRI in his building and they took a scan, and sure enough we knew by that night that it was likely osteosarcoma."

Fortunately, the scan showed they had spotted the cancer early, before it had spread.

When they got home, Paulina and Jason tried to maintain a semblance of normalcy. They had a family dinner and put the kids to bed. But as soon as the kids were asleep, they called their close friends, Chris and Irene, and asked them to come over immediately. "He's a radiation oncologist and she's a pediatrician," Paulina says. They had two girls the same ages as Diego and Mateo and had known the boys all their lives. They came over that night, and took a look at the scans on the computer. After examining the images, they confirmed the bad news: it was almost certainly osteosarcoma.

They could not be certain of the diagnosis until Diego underwent what is called a core-needle biopsy. A doctor takes a long, hollow needle, inserts it into the tumor, and uses it to extract a core of the tissue to test whether it is cancerous.

Chris said they needed to choose carefully which doctor did the procedure because, he told Paulina, "if somebody does a needle biopsy and they don't do it properly, the cancer can spread." Chris's partner in his medical practice had survived childhood cancer and was treated at St. Jude Children's Research Hospital in Memphis, Tennessee—the cancer center founded by the late entertainer Danny Thomas. It is one of the best pediatric cancer hospitals in the country. He arranged for Diego to go to St. Jude for the test and by Monday the Morris family was on a plane to Memphis.

When they walked through the doors of St. Jude, Diego was terrified. Everywhere he looked he saw kids with cancer. "We love going back there now," Jason says, "but when you're uninitiated and you arrive on a campus like this, it's like being on a planet full of cancerous children all of whom are going through some form of treatment. They have no hair, they're in wheelchairs, they're being pulled around in little red wagons, they all have intravenous drips going, and it's terrifying."

"I hadn't been diagnosed yet," Diego says. "Being there and seeing all the other kids who had cancer . . . everyone around me was a patient with cancer. So that makes it very, very scary."

They stayed at St. Jude for ten days. Doctors opened up Diego's knee and took what's called a frozen section—removing some of the tumor and examining it right there on the operating table. After seeing thousands of tumors, they could tell with a high level of certainty whether it was osteosarcoma.

Diego had been told that if the doctors believed it was cancer, they would immediately place a port in his chest while he was still under anesthesia so he would have his chemotherapy administered without having to use a needle.

When he woke up, the first thing he did was look at his mom and dad and ask:

"Did they put the port in?"

"Yes," his parents said.

"So I've got cancer?" Diego cried out.

Jason nearly breaks down recalling the moment. "It's a string of horrible memories that I try not to think about, and as I'm telling you I'm shaking," he says.

A few days later the lab results came in and confirmed the diagnosis. Paulina and Jason had to make some quick decisions. Diego needed ten weeks of chemotherapy to reduce the size of the tumor before he underwent resection surgery to remove it, and then limb-salvage surgery to see if doctors could save his leg. Before 1970 the only way to treat osteosarcoma had been amputation of the affected limb, but today doctors can save the limb in most cases so long as the cancer remains localized.

The doctors at St. Jude encouraged the Morrises to stay in Memphis for both the chemotherapy and the surgeries. But they also told Jason and Paulina that the presurgery chemotherapy was standard for every child who has osteosarcoma, which meant they could also get it back in Phoenix. "We could go to the hospital basically less than a mile from us and he would receive the same treatment and he'd be able to be around his friends and he'd be able to sleep in his own bed at night," Jason says.

Paulina and Jason decided as a family to bring Diego back to Phoenix for the chemo. The whole experience had been overwhelming for the eleven-year-old. In less than a week, he had gone from playing soccer with his friends to a hospital bed in a children's cancer ward fourteen hundred miles from home. He was scared, he was homesick, and he missed his new puppy, Mojo.

"We wanted to be in our home, we wanted to have Diego in his bed as much as possible," Paulina says. "We knew the strength of being at home and having your support system around you."

Little did they know they would soon have to leave that support system behind and uproot their family in order to save their son.

After finishing his chemotherapy at Phoenix Children's Hospital, Diego boarded the flight back to Memphis for his surgery at St. Jude. He now looked like the children who had terrified him on his first visit to the hospital.

"He had lost all his hair; he was walking on crutches," Jason says.

During the flight, Jason noticed that the man in the seat near Diego was chatting him up. Toward the end of the flight, the man came up to Jason and introduced himself.

"Hi, I talked to your son. I understand you're going to St. Jude. It's an amazing place, you couldn't be taking him to a better place. If it's all right with you, I live in Memphis, I'd like to stop by and keep in touch." The man said his name was Joe and Jason gave him his business card. That was just the type of kindness they had encountered in Memphis. It felt like the entire city had embraced the children of St. Jude.

Jason said, "I'm touched, thank you very much." He thought nothing of it.

The next day, Jason's secretary called. "There's a guy named Joe Theismann who called and wants your mobile number," she told him. The man on the plane was the former Washington Redskins quarterback and Super Bowl champion. He was on the board of St. Jude and came to visit Diego and took the family to lunch. For a sports fanatic like Diego, it was one bright moment of happiness in an otherwise devastating time.

Soon, Diego went into surgery. Doctors were able to remove all of the tumor and save his leg. But when the procedure was over, the Morrises got some bad news. The chemotherapy Diego underwent before surgery had not been as effective as his doctors had hoped. Ideally, presurgery chemotherapy kills 90 percent or more of the cancer. In Diego's case, it had reduced the tumor by only 50 percent.

That meant the risk that Diego's cancer could return and spread was high.

When osteosarcoma comes back, it does not usually return at the site of the original tumor. It comes back in the lungs. And once osteosarcoma reaches the lungs, it is highly resistant to chemotherapy. Diego's cancer had already resisted the initial cycle of chemotherapy, so there was a significant risk that even the most extensive chemotherapy alone would not prevent the cancer from returning.

Osteosarcoma has a 70 to 85 percent mortality rate once it has spread.[1]

There had to be something more they could do, Paulina thought.

Back home, the Morrises' friends Chris and Irene had been researching osteosarcoma treatments and one day they called Paulina and Jason with some exciting news. They had found a drug that might be able to help Diego.

"You need to see these studies about this drug, mifamurtide, that is showing some promising results with kids just like Diego," they said.

Mifamurtide (also known as MEPACT or MPT) is a biological therapy that stimulates the immune system to attack cancer. The drug activates large white blood cells called macrophages (which is Greek for "big eaters") and gets them to hunt down, engulf, and devour cancer cells.

To work, mifamurtide has to be given at the same time as postsurgical chemotherapy. The two treatments work in tandem. According to a description of the drug from MD Anderson Cancer Center in Houston, where it was discovered, "The chemotherapy acts like a bomb sent in to destroy the tumor, while MEPACT acts as a special forces unit sent in to clean out any remaining pockets of microscopic disease."[2]

The drug was pioneered at MD Anderson by a doctor named Eugenie Kleinerman. She began studying mifamurtide in 1982 as a young researcher at the National Cancer Institute (NCI) after attending a lecture by a colleague, Dr. Josh Fidler, at a national cancer conference. She sat in the audience, mesmerized, as Dr. Fidler described how he had used mifamurtide to eradicate melanoma cancer in the lungs of lab mice.

"What Dr. Fidler did was create a Trojan horse," Dr. Kleinerman says. "One of the jobs of a macrophage is to get rid of old red cells.

When a red cell becomes old, the macrophage says, 'Oh, old red cells, need to get rid of it.'"

Dr. Fidler had fooled the macrophages into thinking that cancer cells were old red cells. He got them to attack the melanoma cells without harming healthy tissue.

If mifamurtide worked against melanoma, Dr. Kleinerman thought, maybe it would work for osteosarcoma as well.

So she reached out to Dr. Fidler and together they decided to find out. They did a series of laboratory studies that showed, first, that human macrophages responded the same way as mouse macrophages (selectively killing tumor cells and not normal cells) and, second, that mifamurtide stimulated human immune cells to react against osteo-sarcoma cells just as it did against melanoma.

The results were exciting, and armed with this preclinical evidence, they approached the National Cancer Institute about conducting clinical trials in humans. But, Dr. Kleinerman says, the institute was focused on other therapies and was not interested in supporting their work.

In 1984 Dr. Fidler was recruited away by MD Anderson Cancer Center. He asked Dr. Kleinerman to come with him. MD Anderson was ready to support their research.

In 1986 they conducted a phase I clinical trial of mifamurtide in humans, which determined the safety and optimal dose of the drug.

Then in 1988 they conducted a phase II trial of the drug in children with osteosarcoma, which showed improved survival in patients who had not responded to chemotherapy.

Finally in 1993 the drug was ready for a large phase III, multicenter clinical trial. So Dr. Kleinerman joined forces with Dr. Paul Meyers at Memorial Sloan Kettering Cancer Center in New York to conduct a massive phase III trial. They recruited about seven hundred newly diagnosed osteosarcoma patients. It was, Dr. Meyers says, "the largest trial of osteosarcoma ever conducted in the world."

But in the midst of the trial, the drug company that owned mifamurtide, Ciba Geigy (now Novartis), stopped manufacturing the drug. "They decided this is an orphan disease, this is an expensive drug to make, we really don't care about it," Dr. Kleinerman says. Fortunately, another company, Jenner Biotherapies, picked mifamurtide up, allowing it to complete the trial. But then Jenner went out of business—leaving the orphan drug an orphan itself.

Without a sponsor to cover the costs, the results were never fully analyzed. In 2005 Drs. Kleinerman and Meyers published a paper describing the data they had collected up to 2003 and said the results were inconclusive. "The addition of MTP to chemotherapy might improve [event-free survival], but additional clinical and laboratory investigation will be necessary," they wrote.[3]

Mifamurtide, it seemed, had hit a dead end.

A few years later Dr. Meyers got a call out of the blue from Bonnie Mills, the vice president of clinical operations at a company called IDM Pharma. IDM had bought the bankrupt drugmaker, and she had been asked to look through the portfolio of drugs it had acquired to see if there were any with untapped potential.

She had some exciting news: mifamurtide worked.

Dr. Meyers recalls, "She said, 'Did you know that your drug actually statistically significantly improved survival among the patients who got it?' And I said, 'What are you talking about?'"

They had never looked at the survival rates.

Dr. Meyers explains that when you do a clinical trial, before you start, you first develop a detailed plan for how you will analyze the results. The plan for the mifamurtide study called for them to take the first look at survival data once they had observed half of the expected patient deaths. "In other words, if you predict there will be 100 deaths and you've seen 49 deaths, you're not supposed to look at the survival data. If you've seen 62 deaths you're allowed to look at the survival data," Dr. Meyers says.

They had never reached the number of deaths required to trigger an analysis of survival data. "The reason we hadn't seen half of the expected deaths was there were fewer deaths than expected," Dr. Meyers says. "Why were there fewer deaths than expected? Because the drug was *actually working.*"

The company decided to go back and track down patients in the trial and confirm how many had survived. The results were astounding. What they found, according to MD Anderson, was that "MEPACT, when given in conjunction with combination chemotherapy, resulted in a 30% reduction in the mortality rate at eight years after diagnosis, compared to the patients who received chemotherapy alone."[4]

It was the biggest breakthrough in the treatment of osteosarcoma in more than two decades.

"At that point," Dr. Meyers says, "the company said we need to go to the FDA and show them these data and ask for approval for this drug. This is an exciting drug, the first drug to punch the needle in this disease for over twenty years."

The FDA did not share their enthusiasm.

"We went to the FDA and we had *extraordinarily* hostile reception," Dr. Meyers says. "I mean a really nasty, angry, 'Get out of my face, what the hell are you doing here' reception."

Why did the FDA react with such hostility to news of a historic breakthrough in the treatment of a rare, but deadly cancer? "I can only speculate," Dr. Meyers says. "I can tell you that the usual course of action in developing a drug is—before you ever initiate the clinical trial that you want to submit for approval—you go to the FDA and you ask them to review your clinical trial. And [they] say, 'Yes, we agree that your trial design is appropriate, your sample size appropriate, your end points are appropriate, we like the way you've designed this trial.' That never happened because when we began the clinical trial no one had the faintest idea that we would ever be seeking approval for this drug."

In other words, the agency was unhappy because it had not been consulted before the trial began.

The FDA also pointed to the article Drs. Kleinerman and Meyers had published, citing their own words back to them declaring that the results of the trial were inconclusive. "We said, 'But we have new data! Look at our new data!'" Dr. Meyers says. "And they said, 'Go away and don't come back.'"

But the company did come back. It insisted that mifamurtide get a formal hearing before the Oncology Drugs Advisory Committee.

"It was as if we had slapped them in the face," Dr. Meyers says. "What are you doing here? We told you not to come back."

The hearing took place on May 9, 2007.[5] The FDA made a very negative presentation before the committee. "The review team and Division Director find that the Applicant, IDM, has failed to demonstrate that their product . . . provides substantial evidence of efficacy," the FDA declared, adding, "FDA finds that there is not sufficient evidence of a survival advantage for the addition of MTP-PE to the standard chemotherapeutic regimen."[6] Dr. Meyers later learned that the FDA had used the old data as the basis of its presentation—not the new data that showed increased survival rates.

Dr. Kleinerman testified that the FDA was wrong. "This is the first time that we have seen a five-year survival rate approaching 80 percent for patients with nonmetastatic disease, the first improvement in the treatment of osteosarcoma in over twenty years," she told the committee. "If we assume that about 600 children will be diagnosed with osteosarcoma each year, we estimate the use of MTP will save an additional 50 children per year in the United States or 500 children in 10 years. . . . If it is not approved at this time, we will have failed our patients. For every year that MTP's use is delayed, fifty potential avoidable deaths will occur from osteosarcoma. Our patients must have access to this agent," she declared.[7]

Drs. Kleinerman and Meyers brought in patients who had been

cured by mifamurtide to testify. The Sarcoma Foundation of America came to lobby for approval of the drug.

Yet despite their best efforts, the drug was rejected.[8]

"I was extremely depressed," Dr. Kleinerman says.

A few months later, she got a call from IDM. It still believed in mifamurtide and had decided to bring it before the European Medicines Agency (EMA), the European equivalent of the FDA. IDM asked her and Dr. Meyers to help them guide mifamurtide though the approval process in Europe. They agreed.

The process in Europe was completely different. "Each country has two representatives and you walk in the room and it looks like the United Nations," Dr. Kleinerman says. "They're sitting around and viewing computers. So [unlike the FDA] they're viewing the primary data"—including the new survival data the FDA had ignored.

The FDA had given them just a few hours to make their case. By contrast, the European agency put them through three hearings. "They sent a team of auditors to sites around the United States which had participated in a clinical trial including my hospital," Dr. Meyers says. "I had four auditors in my hospital for five days. They were looking at the patients' charts to be sure that the data we wrote down and submitted to the data management center was accurate."

Based on its careful review of the new information and its field investigation of the clinical trial, the EMA determined that mifamurtide was safe and effective. It approved it in 2009 for use in all twenty-seven EU member states as well as Iceland, Liechtenstein, and Norway.[9]

In 2011, after a careful three-year review, mifamurtide was also approved by Britain's National Institute for Health and Care Excellence (NICE), the agency that determines which drugs will be paid for by the government in the United Kingdom. NICE chief executive Sir Andrew Dillon pointed out that while only 150 new cases of osteosarcoma are diagnosed in the United Kingdom each year, "for the small number of patients who benefit from Mifamurtide, the health benefits continue over the rest of their lives, effectively being a cure."[10]

In 2012 mifamurtide received the prestigious Prix Galien Award, the gold medal for pharmaceutical research and development in the United Kingdom. At a gala in London, Professor Sir Michael Rawlins, president of the Royal Society of Medicine, declared, "Apart from its novel mechanism of action—and clear evidence of its clinical effectiveness—the jury were also extremely impressed that such an advance in the management of osteosarcoma represents the first significant change in outcomes in ten to twenty years of managing this disease."

The more Paulina and Jason Morris learned about mifamurtide, the more excited they became. An award-winning drug that could reduce their son's risk of dying by 30 percent, and has been declared a "cure" by the British government?

Mifamurtide seemed perfect for Diego.

The problem was, the drug was still not available in America.

After the EMA approved mifamurtide, a Japanese pharmaceutical company, Takeda, acquired IDM Pharma, and the rights to mifamurtide. Takeda tried to bring the drug back to the FDA for approval. Now that the EMA had endorsed mifamurtide, surely its American counterpart would have to acknowledge the possibility that it had made a mistake and take another look.

"They tried to go to the FDA and [asked them] to re-review the data," Dr. Kleinerman says. "And they refused to re-review the data. They're insisting on another trial." The trial the FDA demanded would require approximately nine hundred patients. There are only about eight hundred new cases of osteosarcoma a year to begin with, so finding nine hundred patients to participate in a *second* large trial for a disease this rare would be next to impossible. The cost was prohibitive. "What the FDA is requiring would cost them $160 million and they just cannot justify that outlay of resources for an orphan disease," Dr. Kleinerman says.

While mifamurtide languishes in a bureaucratic quagmire here in the United States, more and more countries across the world have approved it for use. "It is standard of care in the UK, Spain, Portugal, and Italy," Dr. Kleinerman says. "Israel, everyone is getting it. Korea did another study and they duplicated our findings that there was superior overall survival in patients that got mifamurtide. This summer I'm going to Kazakhstan. It's being launched in Thailand, it's being launched in Colombia, Mexico, Venezuela."

Dr. Meyers is traveling the world as well. "I'm leaving for Argentina on Wednesday to talk to the Argentinean oncologists about the drug. I'm going to Finland in two weeks to talk about the drug." Dr. Meyers does not make a penny from mifamurtide. He does it, he says, because "I believe that the drug works. I believe the drug should be available for every child with osteosarcoma. It's not available in the United States and it doesn't look as if it will ever be available in the United States.

"My strategy is simple," he says. "I plan to get this drug approved in 194 of the 195 countries on earth. At some point the cure rate for osteosarcoma in those countries will exceed the cure rate for the US and people will start to ask questions about why."

Over the years, Dr. Kleinerman has kept up with several of the clinical trial patients she treated in the United States. "In my phase II study, I had one young man whose pediatric oncologist sent him home to die. He was in high school. He's now an orthopedic oncologist at the University of Pittsburgh," she says. Another patient was a young Vietnamese girl whose mother brought her to MD Anderson to be treated. "I was at her wedding ten years ago. I was at her wedding. These are kids that are cured.

"So the tragedy is, US children showed it was effective. It was developed in the United States. A lot of my preclinical work was supported by National Institutes of Health grants. We can no longer get it in this country," she says.

What does she think of the FDA approval process? "I think it is broken," Dr. Kleinerman says. "My experience with the FDA is [like] a saying in my house about men. What are the three things men can never say? 'I was wrong.' 'I'm sorry.' And 'I'm lost.' So I think the FDA cannot say: Perhaps we didn't judge this correctly. Let's take another look. Perhaps we were wrong."

She does not fault the FDA alone. "I also fault my pediatric oncology colleagues, because I think if we would get together and were more vocal and put pressure on the FDA—but everybody is afraid, you know. Well, if I make them mad then my hospital president won't be happy, and I won't get my tenure renewal, or I won't get promoted, the FDA will not put my trial in—you can create a hundred scenarios."

Mifamurtide, she says, is "a drug that has a great safety profile with over 25 years of data. . . . It is adding benefit in terms of survival with good quality of life. I would think you would bend over backward to see how you could get this available for patients in this country."

But it is not available for patients in this country—and that meant Diego Morris would have to go abroad to get the drug he needed to save his life.

PAULINA AND JASON COULD not believe they were unable to get the drug Diego desperately needed—a safe and effective drug in use across the world—here in America. And because he needed to start immediately, at the same time he underwent postsurgery chemotherapy, they had only a brief window to gain access to this life-saving medication.

"We tried everything," Paulina says. "We talked to the drug manufacturer. We talked to our political representatives' offices. We talked to the FDA. We tried every avenue we could think of to get the drug here. Because, like our initial decision of having chemotherapy in Phoenix, we knew the value of being in your own home and having your loved ones around you."

They looked into clinical trials, Jason says, "but all the trials had finished and the FDA had denied approval." They looked into the FDA's "compassionate use" program, but that was a dead end. The FDA had stopped compassionate use of mifamurtide in 2012. So they started looking abroad.

"We contacted the drug company and said, 'Is there anything else going on? Are you testing this somewhere else in the world?'" Jason says. "And they said, 'No we're not testing it somewhere else in the world, because it's being used elsewhere in the world.'" That was when they learned about all the countries where mifamurtide was available.

They kept looking for a way to get it here at home. One option was to get the drug abroad and import it themselves—just like the AIDS activists in the movie *Dallas Buyers Club*. The rep from the drug manufacturer explained it was legal in Mexico and being used routinely by patients. She offered to explore which border city would be closest to them. "They would meet us at the border and we could import it ourselves," Jason says.

At first it seemed like the perfect solution, but the more Jason and Paulina thought about it, the more problems they saw. "This drug has to be kept refrigerated and I was worried: how do we do that?" Jason says. "Secondly, if it was confiscated, what if they didn't refrigerate it? Would I ever get it back? It's about a quarter of a million dollars worth of drugs. So that would be money thrown away if we didn't have the drugs. And then, the last part is I'd need to find somebody to administer it and I wouldn't want to put any of my medical friends at risk and ask them to do that because that's asking them to put their career on the line. So, although it was tempting, that didn't seem like a solution for us."

They quickly came to a stark realization. If they were going to get the drug for Diego, they would have to move to a foreign country.

But where? Jason and Paulina began reaching out to every hospital and clinic across the world they could find that treated patients with mifamurtide. "I called some doctors in Israel and some doctors in Germany and Italy and London," Jason says. The good news was, every clinic they contacted said Diego was welcome.

They weighed the different options. "Israel was appealing, but there are no direct flights between Israel and Arizona. And in addition to worrying about my son's health, I would be worried about the political reality in the Middle East," he said.

Another possibility was Mexico. Irene, their pediatrician friend who had helped diagnose Diego, was born outside Mexico City. She quickly found a hospital there that was treating children with mifamurtide. So Irene, Paulina, and Jason got on a plane to Mexico to investigate.

"The three of us flew there; my husband and I and this doctor," Paulina says. "She interpreted medical Spanish. And the doctors there told us how promising this drug was and they showed us scans, and they showed us basically the drug at work on the children they were using it on. It almost looked like Pac-Man. You could see their own bodies going to work on [the cancer]."

They also spoke to Dr. Meyers at Memorial Sloan Kettering—the doctor who had run the mifamurtide studies with Dr. Kleinerman. Jason asked what he would do if it was his son or grandson.

"I would go," Dr. Meyers told Jason, "I would get it."

That is what they decided too.

"We were down to the wire," Jason says. It was either London or Mexico City. Mexico seemed to make the most sense. Jason would have to commute between his job in Phoenix and wherever Diego went for treatment, and Mexico City was closest to their home in Arizona. But Paulina said, "There was also the issue of interpreting medical conversations and that can be very difficult." And, Jason adds, "I was worried about them living in Mexico City."

Jason had family in England and there was a well-regarded clinic in London that was willing to provide the treatment. It would be much farther from home and a much more challenging commute. But they had a support network there and shared a common language with the doctors who would be treating Diego.

They decided to move to London.

"Thank God we were able to make that decision to make that move," Paulina says. "So many people can't."

The Morrises stayed with Jason's first cousin Jack and his wife, Susan. They were just planning to stay there a few days, until they found an apartment near the hospital. But soon their cousins told them to stop looking and stay with them for the full nine months.

"What will happen to your younger son and when you're in the emergency room or in the hospital?" Jack and Susan asked. "How can you possibly handle this when Jason's going to be back in Phoenix quite a bit? Stay with us and let us take care of you."

"So again, we were blessed," Paulina says. "We had a loving family to stay with. And it was still difficult. It was still terrible to be in another country and be away from our home and my husband, Diego's father, at the worst time of your life."

Diego underwent twenty-one rounds of debilitating chemotherapy. "The oncologist had told us this is going to get rough and you're going to be afraid that you're killing him with this chemotherapy, because it's going to ravage his body," Paulina says. "And it sure did. He didn't have an ounce of hair on him. If you ever meet Diego you'll laugh because he's the hairiest kid! [His skin] was translucent. By the last chemotherapy, the skin was coming off of his hands. It was really frightening."

Paulina and Jason had their doubts plenty of times throughout the chemo. Jason says, "The doctor summed it up well when she said, 'This would kill an adult. Children's cells divide faster and they are a little bit more resilient and so we can do this to a child but we couldn't do this to an adult because it would kill them. Their body couldn't take it.'"

At the same time as Diego underwent chemo, he received forty-eight doses of mifamurtide, getting the immune therapy intravenously twice a week for three months, and then once a week for another six months. His body was a war zone, with the chemo "bomb" going off and the mifamurtide "special forces" hunting down the microscopic cancer cells.

All the time that Diego was undergoing the harrowing treatment, Jason commuted back and forth between London and Phoenix every ten to fourteen days.

"He was ridiculously tired," Paulina says, "as you can imagine because you can't get your body reset."

Whenever Diego was out of the hospital, Jason would try to plan fun things for the family to do together to keep his son's spirits up. One night, he got tickets to a show called *STOMP*, in which performers use sticks, garbage cans, and garbage lids as drums. "It was the loudest show," Paulina recalls, "and we were laughing because Jason was asleep throughout the show."

But the hardest part for Jason was not the exhaustion. It was being five thousand miles away during Diego's many scary emergency room trips.

Their oncologist had warned them that Diego would probably find himself back at the hospital often between treatments. "Your immunities are so low, and it's so dangerous at that point, because your platelets are almost zero and your ability to fight anything is so low that it's a scary time," Paulina says. "There were some emergency room visits that were pretty awful that I don't even like to think about. And my husband had to hear about them long distance and that's very difficult for a parent."

Once Diego woke up in the middle of the night with an uncontrollable nosebleed. "At that point his body couldn't stop the bloody nose. So our cousin Jack got a bucket and his wife got towels. And my younger son was freaking out seeing all the blood. He had been really strong through it all, but at that point he latched on to me saying, 'Please don't go.'"

Diego was terrified. "I was having to tell him, 'It's okay, this is normal, we're going to get you to the hospital.' Jason wasn't there and our cousin was speeding trying to get to the hospital because it was faster that way than trying to wait for an ambulance."

Paulina had called ahead to the hospital, so the nurses and doctors were there waiting and went straight to work on Diego. "They were all trying to stop the bleeding and giving him a transfusion and doing as much as possible. But we were scared. We were scared. I remember telling a nurse that I was doing a lot of praying that night. And she said, 'We all were.'"

Jason says that leaving London—knowing he would not be there for his family at those terrible moments—was almost unbearable. "It was excruciating getting on that plane," he says. "It was the most painful ten hours that I would go through. It was truly miserable. I'd have to gear myself up to get on the plane and then I would spend a lot of time on that plane just lost in time and wishing I didn't have to come back [to Phoenix]."

Even after moving to London, the Morris family never stopped trying to get mifamurtide back home. "We never gave up," Paulina says. "We thought there must be a way to get this drug in the United States. It's America, right? We should be able to get things that are showing promise and that are being approved everywhere else in the world."

She recalls how the doctors, nurses, and patients they met at the clinic were stunned that these Americans had to come to London for treatment. "I can't tell you how many times we heard, 'We cannot believe you're Americans getting care in London. We thought you have everything in terms of medicine and access to everything you can get there,'" Paulina says.

She thought to herself, "You're right, we should be able to get this in the United States."

Little did she know that her young son was about to enter the political arena, and help lead the fight to do just that.

. . . .

WHEN HIS TREATMENT WAS complete, Diego and his family returned to Phoenix. They felt like they were coming home from war. No more rushing to the emergency room in the dark of night. No more ten-hour commutes for Jason or juggling plane and treatment schedules. No more watching chemotherapy ravage their son, as a battle took place inside his body to kill the cancer before it killed him.

Once the chemotherapy stopped, Diego's hair came back thicker than ever and he shot up several inches seemingly overnight. "He started to grow immediately because children don't grow when they're on chemotherapy, because it's stopping the cells from dividing, it's killing everything," Jason says.

Because of the massive dose of chemotherapy Diego received, he needs to get regular tests of his heart and his hearing. "All of the medical staff are amazed at how little impact the amount of chemo he had had on his body," Jason says. "His hearing's great, his heart is wonderful, all of the things that they're most concerned with. So we're blessed."

When she heard about Diego's recovery, Dr. Kleinerman—the MD Anderson doctor who discovered mifamurtide and tried to get it approved here in America—was elated. "It makes all the tough years of frustration I went through with this drug, that's what makes it all worthwhile. All the gray hairs on my head and the broken pieces of glass I've thrown."

Jason and Paulina never forgot how many other people there were who did not have access to drugs like mifamurtide. They were on the lookout for an opportunity to do something to help others. Jason recalled the conversation he had with Dr. Meyers, at Memorial Sloan Kettering, who encouraged them to go to London to get mifamurtide. Jason was so grateful for his guidance and kindness that he asked Dr. Meyers if there was anything they could do to thank him. "He said, 'I don't need anything. But if you can spread the word and help people get access to this drug that would be great.'"

They found that opportunity in 2014 when the Right to Try initiative came to their home state of Arizona.

I had heard about Diego from my Goldwater Institute colleague, Victor Riches, who told me the amazing story of an Arizona boy who nearly died from cancer and whose family had to move to England to find a cure. We knew we needed to reach out to the Morris family and see if they would be interested in helping the Right to Try effort.

The entire family came to our offices for a briefing, and we walked them through the proposed law and how it could help other kids like Diego. Diego said "yes" immediately, but we asked him to take his time and talk it over with his parents. After a few days of careful consideration, we got a call from the Morrises: Diego enthusiastically agreed to become the honorary chairman of the Right to Try initiative in Arizona.

The state legislature had referred the Right to Try act to the voters as a ballot measure in the November 2014 election. Diego became the face of Arizona's Right to Try campaign, giving speeches, doing radio and television interviews, writing letters to the editor, and even cutting a television campaign ad for Prop 303. He movingly spoke at the Goldwater Institute's headquarters, sharing his story and making the case for the Right to Try. When he was finished, there wasn't a dry eye in the house.

Diego could have been doing anything else at that point. He had been through a harrowing ordeal. He had gotten the treatment he needed. He was finally back home and no one would have blamed him if all he wanted to do was just go to school, spend time with friends, get back on the ball field, and try resuming a normal teenage life. But he wanted to help others. He had been through the vale and now he was going back to bring others through as well. I was inspired by his courage. And so were his mom and dad.

"It was so healthy," Paulina says of Diego's decision to get involved with Right to Try. "We watched him become comfortable with telling his story and knowing that there's no shame and there's no need to hide from this—to be actually proud of your strength and what you've overcome and what you've managed to do.

"We were constantly dropping things to work on the campaign," Paulina continues. "And he loved it. He *loved* it. He loved being able to do something positive, to take something that was so negative, so debilitating, such a nightmare, and turn it into something positive."

His efforts paid off. On November 4, 2014, the people of Arizona approved Right to Try by a margin of 78.5 to 21.5 percent. The victory was overwhelming. Thanks in large part to Diego's tireless campaigning, 1,111,850 people pulled the lever in favor.

Diego and his family celebrated on election night and did interviews with the local media. "Two years ago, I had cancer, and my family and I had to go to another country to get an experimental drug that could have possibly saved my life. And luckily I'm here today," Diego told KJZZ news. Now that Prop 303 was law in Arizona, he said, "it will give people the opportunity to not have to go through what we had to go through."[11]

Thanks to Diego, that was true in the state of Arizona. But in much of the rest of the country, Americans still did not have the Right to Try. And this lack of access to cutting-edge medicines is driving many people with terminal illnesses abroad in the search for cures.

While few Americans have heard of Diego Morris, there was someone almost everyone is familiar with who was forced to travel abroad for treatment.

In fact, you may very well have one of his products in your pocket right now.

# 3.

# What Steve Jobs Saw

*How the FDA Stops American Doctors from*
*Using a Proven Cancer Treament*

———

When Paulina Morris first got her son Diego's diagnosis, she sent him into the lobby to play on her iPad while she talked to his doctor—the start of a long journey that would take her family halfway across the world to cure Diego's cancer.

What Paulina did not know at the time was that the man who invented that iPad had taken a similar journey.

For the past two decades, the most respected American doctors in the field of carcinoid and neuroendocrine cancer have been sending their patients to clinics in Rotterdam, the Netherlands; Bad Berka, Germany; and Basel, Switzerland.

They have had to, because the most effective treatment is still not available here in America.

In 2004 Steve Jobs, the founder and CEO of Apple, was diagnosed with a rare cancer in his pancreas called neuroendocrine carcinoma, or NET cancer. According to the Center for Carcinoid and Neuroendocrine Tumors at the Mount Sinai School of Medicine in New York, "About 12,000 cases are diagnosed each year in the United States, and it has been estimated that there are 102,000 people in the country with this slowly progressing malignancy."[1]

Jobs was extremely secretive about his diagnosis and course of treatment, so many of the details are not known to this day. According to news reports, he at first decided against surgery, seeking to treat his cancer with a special diet. Then, according to his biographer Walter Isaacson, Jobs underwent cancer drug therapy that "had grueling side effects. His skin started drying out and cracking."

Finally, Isaacson writes, "in his quest for alternative approaches, he flew to Basel, Switzerland, to try an experimental hormone-delivered radiotherapy . . . developed in Rotterdam known as Peptide Receptor Radionuclide Therapy"—or PRRT for short.[2]

It's a complicated name, but the concept behind it is actually quite simple.

The cells in NET cancer tumors have a receptor on the surface which binds to a hormone (or peptide) in the body called somatostatin. In the 1980s researchers developed a laboratory-made version of this peptide called octreotide. When it is injected into the bloodstream, it travels through the body, finds the cancer cells, and attaches itself to them. It is used principally for diagnostic purposes (as part of what is called an OctreoScan that helps doctors locate tumors in the body) though it is also used as a treatment because the peptide has some cell-inhibiting impact.[3]

In PRRT, the therapy Steve Jobs underwent, doctors turn that diagnostic tool into a highly effective cancer killer by adding a small amount of radioactive material to the peptide before injecting it into the bloodstream. This turns the peptide into a radiopeptide, which not only finds and attaches itself to the cancer cells but then delivers a high dose of radiation directly to the tumors, destroying them.

According to Dr. Richard Warner, director of Mount Sinai's NET cancer center, "The receptor is like a magnet and this [radiopeptide] is like a piece of iron filing. And so this radioactive pharmaceutical agent is injected into the bloodstream . . . and anywhere that a neuroendo-crine tumor having the receptors is located . . . it attracts this material and . . . it gives internal radiation to the tumor."

The beauty of PRRT, he says, is that it can find and kill tumors that are so tiny that doctors cannot find them on a scan. Any NET cancer cell—however small or well hidden in the body it may be—will attract the radiopeptide like a magnet and thus irradiate itself.

PRRT not only hunts down hidden tumors; it also allows doctors to treat tumors that are inoperable because they are embedded in vital organs. It is extremely safe, Dr. Warner says, because "the range of the radioactive rays that it emits is very short, so it doesn't irradiate adja-cent structures. But it does irradiate the tumors to which it's attracted and thereby wounds or kills them by radiation." The radioactive mate-rial is flushed out of the patient's system in a few days.

PRRT is not a cure. The tumors eventually come back, and when they do the process must be repeated. But with multiple treatments, PRRT can beat back NET cancers and add not just weeks or months, but many years to the lives of patients.

It is unknown what impact the treatment had on Jobs, who died in October 2011. But studies show that PRRT has extended the lives of many thousands of other cancer patients. Indeed, it is far more effec-tive at killing NET cancers than chemotherapy.

A 2010 study in Rotterdam found that chemotherapy slowed the progression of NET cancers by less than eighteen months. By contrast, when patients received PRRT using the two most common radioactive agents—Y-90 and Lu-177—they beat back the cancer far longer. In PRRT using Y-90, the treatment slowed their cancer progression for thirty months—a year longer than chemotherapy. Lu-177 was even more effective. It slowed cancer progression for forty months—almost two full years longer than chemotherapy.[4]

Two more years is a lot of time—and some patients can turn that into decades by repeating the treatment. Not only does it buy dying patients more time than chemotherapy; it gives them a much better quality of life. Chemotherapy often has debilitating side effects, because the treatment indiscriminately damages both healthy and cancerous tissues. But according to the Society of Nuclear Medicine and Molecular Imaging, "Radiopeptides are highly selective in their ability to damage neuroendocrine tumor cells, while limiting radiation exposure to healthy tissue. As a result, PRRT typically has milder side effects compared with chemotherapy."[5]

PRRT is safer, has fewer side effects, and is more effective than chemotherapy—which is why, over the past two decades, it has become the standard of care in Europe. Dr. Tom O'Dorisio, a professor of medicine at the University of Iowa and one of the leading NET cancer specialists in America, says that when PRRT was first introduced "all of Europe went bananas with it. Since 1996, every country has had this treatment."

Every country, that is, except the United States.

To this day—despite its widespread use, high success rate, and strong safety profile—PRRT is still not approved for use in the United States. Dr. O'Dorisio and his wife, Dr. Sue O'Dorisio, work as a team at their University of Iowa clinic, treating patients and conducting cancer research. He says, "We, for the first time, just got permission about two days ago from the FDA to do the trial, which is the very same treatment that they've been doing since 1996 in Europe."

The FDA has actually approved *half* of the treatment. Octreotide—the peptide that finds and attaches itself to cancer cells—has been approved by the FDA since the 1980s.

But the FDA does not allow doctors in America to attach the radioactive materials to the peptide that actually destroy the cancer.

This is like giving our military permission to use drones to track down terrorists—just as long as they don't attach a warhead with a bomb that will actually kill them.

If that were not bad enough, the story gets even worse. While the FDA forces American doctors to use the antiquated OctreoScan pioneered in the 1980s—which cannot find many smaller tumors—doctors in Europe are using an advanced high-resolution gallium scan, which is far more effective. The gallium scan uses a radiological material called gallium-68, which is—you guessed it—not approved by the FDA.

Dr. Warner says the gallium scan is "ten times more sensitive" than the FDA-approved OctreoScan. Dr. O'Dorisio says the old scan "sensitivity-wise is kind of like looking through my cataracts," whereas the gallium scan is like looking "through a very precise magnifying glass." The gallium scan, which has been used in Europe for many years, has just been permitted on a clinical trial basis in a few other locations in the United States. One of those is Mount Sinai, Dr. Warner's hospital. But, he says, "We're not allowed to charge for it and we're having problems funding it, because we have to pay for every patient. . . . It costs us about $3,800 for each scan that we do. We're going to run out of money pretty soon."

So most Americans with NET cancers cannot get the most accurate scan to find their tumors, or the most effective treatment to kill those tumors.

So what do these Americans do to save their lives?

Like Diego Morris and Steve Jobs, many go to Europe.

Dr. Tom O'Dorisio says he has personally sent almost 490 patients to the University of Basel Hospital in Switzerland. He says that most of his patients don't have the same resources as Steve Jobs and can't afford to go abroad.

Here's my dilemma, and this is a monster dilemma, and that is that people of means can go. But people who have the same degree of disease, they have glass eyes stare back at you [when you tell them how much it costs]. There's no way they can afford to go for $12,000 per treatment let alone cost for travel. . . . And not just one treatment. They're nine weeks apart and they are anywhere from two to three initially and then three more down the road. So you're talking about an enormous amount of money. And that's the part that's been so ethically tough for me.

In a small number of cases, he is able to convince insurers to cover at least part of the cost. But most patients have to pay for the treatment out of pocket.

His wife, Dr. Sue, says the dilemma is hardest when the patients are children. "Not everybody, and particularly parents, have the resources [to travel abroad]. Usually, with a child, one of them has to quit their job to be able to take care of the child who's sick. And then for both of them to be able to quit their job and take the child over there, that's—I mean it's heroic but not everybody can do it."

At the other end of the spectrum, Dr. Tom says, are the older patients who are retired and on fixed incomes. "The other bad, tragic thing is many of these patients come due at an age when they're in Medicare. And absolutely Medicare will not pay."

Dr. Warner has faced the same dilemma. "I've had literally dozens of patients that I've sent to Europe. . . . And they require four treatments at roughly six-week intervals. So you can figure out what it costs. And of course, being out of the country, it's not covered by anybody's insurance.

"I have a patient waiting to go right now who's trying to get contributions from her friends and other people to cover her treatment . . . she doesn't have the money," he says. "I can think of one fellow who unfortunately died because he couldn't afford it."

What is it like to tell patients their only hope of survival is to get a treatment abroad that they cannot afford and is not covered by insurance?

"It's intolerable," Dr. Warner says. "It really disturbs me and I hate to be in a position where I have to explain that or tell that to people. It makes me feel impotent."

So why is this treatment still not available in America? "The FDA wouldn't accept the data from Europe and required everything to be done all over again here like rediscovering the wheel," Dr. Warner says. "It's been accepted in just about every major country in Europe where it's being widely used. Those of us who are involved and have had patients that were treated know that it's a good treatment and that it does work in 82 percent of the cases, which is a very good statistic."

The man who receives many of the patients referred from America is Dr. Damian Wild, the director of nuclear medicine at the University Hospital of Basel in Switzerland. He says his hospital does about fifty treatments a year for Americans. Asked if the treatment should be available to them at home, he does not hesitate: "Of course it should be, yes.

"We treat American patients; that's not a problem. We like to treat them," he adds. "But of course for many Americans it's a hassle. It's a relatively long trip to Europe and not all of those patients are in very well shape. And so traveling is a hassle for most of those patients."

One patient who learned this firsthand was Lindsey Miller. Before she passed away in May of 2014, she documented her experiences fighting NET cancer on a blog she called *I Am a Liver*. Here is how she described her trip in May 2013 to get treated at a hospital in Germany:

Many many many months ago when I imagined that day far, far in the future that I would (probably) have to travel overseas to seek the famed PRRT treatment for my cancer, I imagined that it would be (secretly) exciting to go to Europe for treatment. That I would get treatment one day and be out eating pretzels and drinking beer the next. I imagined that I would beg my parents to take me to Paris or Prague or Berlin or Amsterdam beforehand, you know, while we were in the area. I imagined I would be wearing heels—isn't that what fabulous European women wear?

Now that the day is today, I am not not excited. I had imagined I would be feeling much better before I left. I have been laying low in my living room for weeks and now i'm supposed to be ready to hop on a plane to fly halfway across the world? I'm not sure i'm up for this; but I have to be, because my tumors are growing and doing crazy things (like causing my legs to swell up) and I need to do something to take care of them. Contrary to my imagination, I will be in the hospital in Germany all week, not eating pretzels or drinking beer. The forecast says rain. I don't have the energy for much sight-seeing. I can't fit into any of my shoes. My suitcase doesn't have room for heels next to all my stretchy pants, compression stockings, prescription bottles, and lung drainage bottles.

In truth, I will be happy when the ordeal is over.[6]

It is shameful that her government put her through such an ordeal. She also wrote movingly for the *Huffington Post* about her struggle to raise money for her treatments.[7] She conducted three successful fund-raising campaigns at a medical crowdfunding site called Give Forward.com that raised about $23,000—enough to put a dent in her medical expenses, but not to cover them.

"The cost is unfathomable," she wrote. "Steve Jobs is rumored to have tried the same treatment at another site in Basel, Switzerland. Presumably, he had no trouble affording it."

And what about the Americans who cannot find the money to go to Europe?

"There's no other FDA-approved treatment," Dr. Tom O'Dorisio says. "Chemotherapy bounces off of these tumors because they're so slow. They're so slow that chemo doesn't work. So all we have is octreotide and people become resistant to the octreotide over time. I turn it upside down. I have tricks that I've learned along the way [to help keep the cancer at bay], but it doesn't hold them. And then people die."

Since there are no other options that can improve survival, Americans often have to spend their life savings to go abroad. That's what happened to Kenneth Jolley, a sixty-four-year-old Vietnam veteran living in Allen, Oklahoma. According to the *Daily Oklahoman*, Jolley was diagnosed in 2011 with stage-four neuroendocrine carcinoid cancer, which had spread to his liver, lung, and chest. His doctors at the Oklahoma City Veterans Administration Medical Center told him there was little he could do but "wait and watch."[8]

Jolley says, "I was classified as Stage 4 and the VA absolutely had no treatment for it. In fact they told me to go home and get my affairs in order."

The Department of Veterans Affairs (VA) offered to pay for palliative care.

That didn't suit this military veteran. "I am not a quitter—I battle," he said. "And I will give up when they put me six feet under."

So he got a second opinion at Vanderbilt University Medical Center in Nashville, where a doctor told him that the best course of treatment was PRRT—but that he would have to travel to Germany to get it. The VA refused to pay for treatment in Europe and so did his insurers. So he was forced to use his retirement savings and borrow money to cover the costs. "Mortgaged everything to the hilt," he says. He traveled to Bad Berka, Germany, three times, at a cost of over $50,000.

The trips were grueling. "When you're looking at an eleven-hour flight three days after you've been treated and this makes you extremely nauseated, you are so miserable by the time you get back here in the States. Every trip, even with medical papers, you spend anywhere from an hour and a half to three hours in Customs trying to get through because you're radioactive."

And after three courses of therapy he could not get in America, Jolley underwent a gallium scan as part of a clinical trial at the National Cancer Institute—which revealed the treatment worked. His existing tumors had shrunk by 42 percent.

When he returned to Oklahoma, he found a clinic in Houston that was conducting a clinical trial of PRRT that was authorized by the FDA. Surely the VA would pay for that, he thought. Wrong. The VA refused, even though at $45,000 the treatment cost less than six months of the palliative care the VA had agreed to cover. His private insurer also refused to pay for the treatment because it is investigational. So he had to pay for it with loans from family and friends and donations he's been able to scrounge up.

"I managed to pay for the first one," he told the *Daily Oklahoman*. "I have no idea how I'm going to pay for the second, but the Lord will provide a way."

When his six-year-old granddaughter, Emerson, heard that Papa Ken was struggling to pay for his medicine, she told her mom: "Well, if I save my allowance for two months, I will give it to him, and then he will have enough money to get better." She saved up forty dollars for her beloved Papa Ken's treatment.

Eventually, after years of fighting, he finally got the VA to relent and pay for his treatment in Houston. "I had exhausted all my funds," he says. "I'm still paying the balance on my treatments in Europe."

Still, even though he's broke, he says he's lucky. "So many people don't have even the resources I have, and they can't just jump on a plane and go to Europe. It's hard to take. As a veteran, it was hard to swallow.

"If [it weren't for] this treatment, I would not be here today," he says.

Is this any way for America to treat a veteran fighting a terminal cancer diagnosis?

The clinical trial Ken Jolley joined was run by Dr. Ebrahim Delpassand, the head of the Excel Diagnostics & Nuclear Oncology Center in Houston, the first research facility in the United States to receive authorization to initiate this much-needed therapy.

Jolley was lucky he could get into the trial when he did. "FDA has just come to me and said that you need to stop this," Dr. Delpassand says. "FDA is allowing us to continue treatment for the previously enrolled patients, but we cannot enroll any new patients at this point. And this is a major disappointment to our patients, to their family members, because really there's no other option here until the drug is commercially available."

Why did the FDA shut down his trial? Dr. Delpassand says, "They said that this therapy has a lot of side effects and it does not. [They said] it doesn't have a meaningful clinical response which, again, that's another really wrong conclusion. The reason that they say this is they don't consider a 'stable disease' as response in these progressive patients. I mean these were patients that the physicians they were giving them three months, six months to live. . . . And now our drug is making them stable for two years, thirty months, [and] FDA doesn't look at it as a response."

Dr. Delpassand says that "this drug has been in use in Europe for a long time, [but] what was lacking was a randomized trial actually, which is considered the gold standard in the scientific way in looking at the effectiveness of this drug." He says that a European company called Advanced Accelerator Applications[9] is now conducting such a trial in Europe and the United States. The trial began recruiting patients in 2012 and completed enrollment in February 2015.

Delpassand says that it will be at least two years before the trial is completed. In other words, by the time the treatment is finally approved in America—*if* it is finally approved in America—it will be two decades after it first went into widespread use in Europe.

Meanwhile, European doctors are already developing the next generation of PRRT treatments. Dr. Tom O'Dorisio says that researchers at the University Hospital in Basel, Switzerland, have developed a new technique he compared to a "broken key."[10]

Dr. Wild, the director of nuclear medicine in Basel, who helped pioneer the new technique, explains that he and his colleagues have found a way to "bend the key of the synthetic hormone so that now it jams longer in the lock. Furthermore more keys can jam in the lock. And so apparently now that a higher number of keys stay longer in the membrane of the tumor cell, it's apparently better than the currently used key that carries the radiopeptide. This results in a several times higher accumulation of radioactivity on the tumor cell."

"It is a big breakthrough," Dr. O'Dorisio says. But that breakthrough is not coming to America anytime soon. In Europe, he says, "they are putting other treatments on top of the ones we don't have" while here in America "we're still flopping around like fish trying to get" the old treatment.

So what is the solution?

Dr. Delpassand thinks he knows. He points to the Right to Try laws. He says,

> The Right to Try Act essentially says that that is the decision between patient and their physician for the investigational drug. Of course the drug should have had phase I trial showing the basic safety of the drug. But after that, it is between physician and the patient. And patients with terminal diseases, which cancer is considered a terminal disease, they can request investigational drugs and their physicians can provide it to them.
>
> Going through the FDA process, one, is extremely expensive and two, is extremely lengthy. And here there are many patients that they don't have that kind of timing in their life. They need the medication much earlier. So something like having the Right to Try Act I think helps in those situations.
>
> If that law passes [in Texas] we don't need FDA's blessing on this. We can go ahead and treat the patients.

A few weeks after he said that, the Texas legislature passed and Governor Greg Abbot signed Right to Try into law in Texas. At this writing, Dr. Delpassand is working with lawyers and Texas officials to clear the way to providing the treatments under the new law.

Another doctor who is preparing to treat patients permitted by Right to Try is Dr. Eugene Woltering, professor of surgery and neuroscience and director of surgical research at Louisiana State University Health Sciences Center/Ochsner in Kenner, Louisiana. On May 30, 2014, Louisiana governor Bobby Jindal signed Right to Try into law. "This is . . . about individual freedom and liberty," Jindal said. "If individuals facing terrible diseases want to try something, why should the government stop them from doing that?"[11]

Will Woltering use the new law to offer PRRT at Ochsner Medical Center? "Oh, absolutely. Yeah, we're doing the Right to Try," he says. "I mean we are just ready to flip the on switch and start treating people," he says.

As soon as the law passed, he says, "I sat down with the Attorney General's Office through my connections at LSU, where I'm a professor. Met with the chancellor, met with the dean. Everybody was really excited. The Ochsner system and the LSU system has agreed with me, and the Attorney General's Office has agreed with me."

All that is left, he says, "is to get the local bureaucrats who have to sign off on nuclear pharmacy regulations at the hospital level.

"The minute we get the sign-off we'll be on top of this like white on rice," he says.

He simply needs to put the radiological agent onto the FDA-approved peptide, octreotide—to effectively attach the warhead onto the drone.

Doing that is easy, he says, "because it requires so little drug. You're hooking the blimp to a grain of rice. The radioactivity is the big kahuna and the amount of peptide that it takes to do a therapeutic dose is micrograms. . . . So for $25,000 worth of drug you can make enough drug to treat a hundred people."

He expects to be up and running this year.

"I'm a huge advocate" of Right to Try laws, he says. "I mean I think that this ought to be the wave of the future. People who have no other options need to be given options."

He says he tried working with the FDA to allow PRRT at his clinic.

"We have people who are dying who maybe have a year to live at the max, having failed all conventional therapies," he says. "And so we go to the FDA and we say we would like to treat somebody with PRRT. And their argument is, 'Yeah, but five years from now they could develop renal failure.' And I'm going, 'These people would be happy to go to their own funeral five years from now rather than a year from now.' And they go, 'No, that's not the way it works.'"

The way it works now in Louisiana is that patients with a year to live will finally have the Right to Try.

Dr. Woltering's message to the FDA? "Quit regulating and micromanaging every little piece of information that we have. Be working with the docs who are trying to take care of patients, not working against them."

Drs. Tom and Sue O'Dorisio also support Right to Try laws. "That's the system that's in place in Europe, which is why Europe is ahead of us," Dr. Sue says. "Any physician in Europe is allowed to treat a patient on a personal basis if they think it's clinically indicated."

Dr. Tom agrees. "We try to play by the rules," he says, "but this is a new rule. I think it's very exciting. I think if there was a Right to Try, you know . . . I'd be not ambivalent but say it could be very valuable if it was carried forward in a systematic way."

The fact that Americans with deadly cancers have to travel abroad to get treatments that should be available right here at home is appalling. Right to Try will soon help these patients get access to these treatments without having to cross an ocean. It puts the decision back where it belongs—between doctor and patient.

Right to Try it is only part of the solution. Dr. Woltering can move forward so quickly because, with PRRT, he does not have to convince a drug company to provide the product. But today, FDA rules discourage drug manufacturers from providing investigational drugs to dying patients even under its own compassionate use program.

We need a system that encourages drug companies to rescue dying patients. We need a system that moves quickly to approve safe treatments. And we need a system that can help patients *now*. It's time for the powers that be to take a lesson from Steve Jobs and the folks at Apple:

"Think Different."

# 4.

# Making Medical Miracles

*The Cutting-Edge Cancer Killers*
*You Can't Get Yet*

————

While Americans must travel abroad for proven cancer treatments blocked by the FDA, doctors here in North America are pioneering the next generation of cancer treatments, with cures and therapies that were once unimaginable.

But most Americans can't get access to these treatments either—unless they are among the 3 percent of cancer patients who qualify for and are able to participate in a clinical trial. For the rest, they must wait for years, sometimes a decade or more, for the government to approve these revolutionary therapies. That is time most people with a terminal diagnosis don't have.

Speeding access to these treatments is why Cancer Treatment Centers of America came to the Goldwater Institute in the first place—and the reason we launched the Right to Try.

ON A CLEAR MORNING in June 2013 Stacy Erholtz woke up with a mission: this was the day that she was going to finally kill Evan.

Make no mistake, Evan had it coming. He had put a hole in Stacy's head the size of a golf ball. And he was getting more aggressive with each passing day. If Stacy didn't kill him now, he was going to kill her for sure. Time was running out.

Stacy had a plan. She was going to kill Evan by exposing him to a deadly virus. The virus would overwhelm Evan's internal defenses, and then begin replicating itself inside him, until his cells began to explode and he died.

Sound horrible? Don't be alarmed. Stacy is no serial killer. She is a fifty-year-old mom from Pequot Lakes, Minnesota, who is fighting multiple myeloma—a deadly blood cancer that attacks bone marrow.

"Evan" is her brain tumor.

Evan grew under her forehead and pressed so hard on her skull that he finally broke through the bone, leaving a large lump exposed. Stacy's kids gave him the name.

They wanted Evan dead too.

Evan was not alone. Stacy had tumors growing on her collarbone, on her sternum, and up and down her spine. "On the scans, I lit up like a Christmas tree," she says.[1] She had been fighting this disease for ten years, but no matter what treatments she tried, her cancer kept coming back with a vengeance. She was dying and running out of options.

"For the longest time, my local doctors couldn't figure out what was wrong with me," she said in an interview on the Mayo Clinic website.[2] When Stacy first went to her physician complaining of chronic fatigue and neck pain, she received a prescription for Celebrex, an anti-inflammatory drug. It had no effect. Her symptoms got worse. She experienced random vomiting and threw her back out. Her tongue became swollen and she got sores in her mouth. She developed bumps and bruising around her eyelids, lost fifty pounds, and twice underwent surgery for carpal tunnel syndrome. She was constantly exhausted. She grew so tired she had to crawl up the stairs to get to her bedroom. One day, she slipped on the ice and cracked her spine.

Finally, she went to an internist, who referred her to an oncologist.

He did multiple tests, including a bone-marrow biopsy, and finally gave her the correct diagnosis: multiple myeloma.

By that point, Stacy was too sick to be devastated. She just wanted to know what was wrong and find a course of treatment. She had two bone-marrow transplants, which did not work. Finally, she was sent to the Mayo Clinic in Rochester, Minnesota, where Dr. Stephen Russell, took over her treatment.

"She was just forty-nine when she came to the clinic with relapsing myeloma about nine months after her most recent bone-marrow transplant," Dr. Russell says. "She had a large sort of egg-sized tumor growing out of her left forehead. We did a CT scan and found that she had four other tumors in her body as well as that one that were all very hot on the CT scan. We also put a needle in her bone marrow . . . and we found that that was diffusely infiltrated by myeloma cells."

At Mayo, Stacy underwent all the standard government-approved treatments. She had her first stem-cell transplant. At first it appeared to work, but then the cancer came back. She tried a variety of novel antimyeloma drugs. The effect was the same—temporary improvement, after which her cancer always returned.

One day when Stacy was watching the news she saw her physician, Dr. Russell, discussing exciting new research he was doing using the measles virus to combat multiple myeloma. The idea was to administer a version of the measles vaccine that most Americans get as children, except the virus is given in much higher doses and is genetically engineered to kill cancer cells.

The virus would enter the bloodstream, bind itself to cancer tumors, and use them as hosts—turning them into machines to replicate itself and eventually destroying the tumors. Any remaining cancer cells in the bloodstream would now have the measles vaccine's genetic imprint, which would trick the body into thinking that they are measles virus. "Then the immune system can come in and mop up the residue," Dr. Russell explained.[3]

Stacy listened transfixed. She was convinced that this was the treatment that would save her. "From that point forward," Stacy says, "I pestered him at every appointment."[4]

The use of viruses to fight cancer was nothing new. Doctors have long used viruses against cancer by injecting them directly into individual tumors to shrink and destroy them.

But what Dr. Russell was doing was different. In this revolutionary treatment, the virus would be injected not into the tumor, but into the patient's *bloodstream*. Once infused, it would conduct a search-and-destroy mission—hunting down and killing cancer that had spread throughout the body.

This had never been tried before. If it worked, it would be the first time in medical history that viral therapy had been successfully deployed against distributed, metastasized cancer in a human being.

Dr. Russell chose the measles virus because, he says, it is extremely safe. Billions of doses have been given to children over the course of many decades.

"We were very concerned about safety and we wanted the virus that we worked with to be one that was absolutely not going to cause risks to the human population or to the treated patient," he says. Measles was the obvious choice because "natural measles infection in America is associated with 0.01 percent mortality and we know that most of the population is immune to measles virus." There was no chance of unleashing the Andromeda strain.

Another advantage, he says, is that the measles virus is capable of infecting blood cells—which makes it perfectly suited for treating blood cancers like multiple myeloma. Moreover, while most Americans are inoculated against measles as children, patients with multiple myeloma have compromised immune systems and tend lose their measles immunity—which means they have no protection against the measles virus.

Viruses are particularly effective cancer killers because a virus is about a thousand times smaller than a cell, Dr. Russell says, so it can bind itself to the cell, take over the cell, and then turn into a factory for the production of new viruses.

"We call viruses 'pirates of the cell,'" he explains.

Viruses are also easy to transform. First, doctors can adapt the virus to kill cancer by training it and evolving it in a culture. Second, they can manipulate its genetic code—removing genes that attack healthy tissue and inserting genes that attack cancer.

The genome of the measles virus, Dr. Russell says, has only six genes, so "we can go in and we can change the genes at will and then re-create a virus with altered genes."

To treat multiple myeloma, Dr. Russell and his team trained the virus in cultures to attack multiple myeloma cells. Then they stitched a new gene into the measles virus that would allow them to follow its fate once it was released into the body.

"One of the scary things about giving a virus as a therapy is that you give it and it's going to grow in the patient and it's going to move around the body," he says. "And our hope is that the virus just specifically attacks tumor wherever it is in the body. But how do we actually keep tabs on that? We can't give the patient a virus and then come and biopsy every tissue every five minutes."

So to keep tabs on the virus, Dr. Russell added a genetic tracer to it. "We can give a virus that has a kind of 'snitch' in it, that allows us to see where it's up to and do an imaging study and see where in the body is this infection now taking place."

The "snitch" he added to the measles virus also made it a more effective cancer killer. "The gene that we put in . . . causes radioactive iodine to concentrate in the virus infected cells, which enhances the ability of the virus to kill the cells," he says. "So it's a way of delivering radioactivity to the site of tumor growth. We call that radio viral therapy. We add the radioactive iodine to the viral therapy and basically increase the potency. The two together are better than either alone."

If his theory was right, the measles virus would kill the cancer in two stages.

"The first we call the oncolytic phase when the virus is just killing the tumor cells directly by infecting them," Dr. Russell says. "The cancer cell becomes a slave to the virus when it's infected, and just makes numerous copies of viruses to the expense of everything else. So it stops taking care of itself and it therefore dies."

The second is called the immune phase. Cancer cells that survive the initial attack by the virus are then targeted by the immune system. The virus essentially paints a target on the cancer cells, which makes the immune system think they are a measles infection and go after them and kill them.

"So [the cancer] dies either because the virus kills it or because the immune system recognizes there's a problem and kills it," Dr. Russell says. "It's really a timing question of whether the immune system will kill the cell before the virus kills it."

Radio viral therapy seemed perfect for Stacy. But when she first applied for the clinical trial, she was rejected. Dr. Russell explained to Stacy that she did not qualify because she had not exhausted all the existing FDA-approved treatments.

"You have to be the biggest loser first," she says. "I needed to fail every type of treatment available before I could qualify for the study."[5]

So she had another stem-cell transplant and tried the remaining available myeloma drugs. It took about eighteen months, but by May 2013 she had undergone every possible treatment. Nothing had worked. So she was finally admitted into the trial.

Those delays may have actually saved her life.

When the FDA allowed Dr. Russell to begin his first human trials, the agency required that he start at extremely low doses of measles vaccine. "They then insist that you design the trial such that you start from a guaranteed safe dose," he says.

The FDA, in its wisdom, determined that a safe dose was one million infectious units—a dose Dr. Russell knew would not be enough to beat back the cancer.

"We knew from our mouse studies that we'd have to give a minimum of a thousand times that dose to have a hope of seeing anything in terms of efficacy," he says.

What that meant was that the patients who volunteered for the early stages of the trial hoping for a cure stood no chance of clinical benefit until the FDA allowed Russell to get to that top dose.

"I just think that it's fundamentally wrong," Dr. Russell says. "I think if somebody has reached the end of their viable options, and wants to try something experimental, they don't want to try a homeopathic dose. They are prepared to take a risk. But the rules imposed by FDA say, 'Well, tough, you can't do that.'"

He adds, "I'm not criticizing the guys at FDA, okay? I suppose what I'm criticizing is the policy under which they labor. What they're told is safety first. And so they're not given the option of looking at the balance between the risk and the benefit, and the ethical considerations behind whether a patient should be given an opportunity."

As a doctor treating patients, he says, "I struggle with that. I certainly know if I had terminal cancer, and I wanted to try a virus, I definitely wouldn't want to try if I was getting a dose that wasn't going to work."

By the time Stacy was allowed to join the trial, the FDA had approved a dose containing one hundred billion infectious units. That was enough measles vaccine to inoculate ten million people—and, more important, enough virus to have a chance at being effective against her cancer.

On June 5, 2013, Stacy arrived at Saint Mary's Hospital in Rochester, Minnesota, for what was supposed to be a thirty-minute viral infusion. She was about to become only the second person in the world to receive such a massive dose.

Dr. Russell inserted a needle into her forearm and the virus began to slowly drip down into her veins. At first she was fine, but five minutes into the treatment, Stacy developed a terrible headache.

"We had to stop it," Dr. Russell says. "It was the worst headache she'd ever had." They treated her headache and asked if she wanted to call off the treatment, but Stacy insisted on going forward. "After it settled she said, 'Right, I want to do this,'" Dr. Russell says. So they resumed the infusion.

It took an hour to get all of the measles virus into her system. "She was fine for a couple of hours," Dr. Russell says, "and then she started rigoring. Her temperature went up very high. It was about 104, 105."

Her immune system was kicking in, responding to the measles invasion. She passed out from the pain.

The next morning, Stacy opened her eyes and looked around her hospital room.

She felt perfectly fine.

So good, in fact, that she was able to check out of the hospital that day and walk across the street to her hotel. One day of feeling awful and the next she was better. That had never happened with any of the other treatments. They had all either required long hospital stays or sapped her energy for extended periods.

But would the treatment work?

A day and a half after her infusion, Stacy told Dr. Russell that Evan had started to soften and had begun shrinking. And within a few weeks, Evan was gone.

After six weeks, a scan showed no sign of disease anywhere in her body. None at all.

All the other tumors were gone.

"There was no evidence of any cancer that we could detect," Dr. Russell says. Stacy was in full remission.

They had made medical history. It was the first time that a patient with cancer spread throughout the body had gone into complete remission through intravenous viral therapy.

Unfortunately, the other patient in the trial didn't have the same lasting results. The virus shrank the cancer, but it came back after nine months.

"I think if we had been able to give a bigger dose, we might have gotten a better outcome in the second patient," Dr. Russell said.[6]

The lesson is that "number one, you need a really big dose and, number two, the patient needs not to have an antibody to the virus."[7] He is now studying ways to break down the body's immune system before treatment in hopes that the treatment can be harnessed for people who do have measles immunity.

Like the ax murderer in a bad horror movie, nine months after Stacy's treatment, Evan made one final attempt to return.

When Evan reappeared, Dr. Russell ran all the diagnostic tests and scans and, he says, "We couldn't see any evidence of cancer elsewhere." It was just Evan. So Dr. Russell finished him off with a dose of radiation therapy. He has not returned since and Stacy has no other signs of cancer.

Evan was dead. And Stacy was alive.

"I saw her back a couple weeks ago," Dr. Russell says. "She's now twenty-one months out from the viral therapy and she remains in complete remission. And you know, she just is on top of the world. She says this is the best therapy she's ever had because all other myeloma therapy, she's kind of had to stay on long term and they've really impacted her quality of life in a negative way. Whereas with this, she's been off all therapy and she just kind of feels like she got her life back."

Dr. Russell says Stacy is now focused on helping other patients achieve the same remission she has.

"She keeps on pestering me, saying, 'When are you going to actually achieve the same thing in another patient?'" he says. "And we haven't yet done that. But that's our obsession now . . . [to] turn this into a reproducible reliable outcome for patients who are treated with the virus."

Since word of Stacy's recovery spread, Dr. Russell has been inundated with requests by patients seeking the same treatment.

He has given the treatment to a number of patients outside the clinical trial on a compassionate use basis. "Because this whole thing is owned by Mayo Clinic and there isn't a company at the moment in control of it, then it's sort of a Mayo Clinic decision. And so we have our mantra—the needs of the patient come first."

He says, unfortunately, for most of the patients the treatment did not work.

"Those individuals have been people with very high disease burden and it hasn't been the answer that they were looking for," he says.

However, the process of attempting to save these late-stage patients through compassionate use taught him some critical lessons. "What we think at the moment is that probably it's going to be very important the amount of myeloma that the patient has in their body and the stage of the disease," he says. "Because we did try to treat people who had very, very advanced myeloma—who had so much disease in their body that they probably had not long at all to live. And we found that the virus was not able to impact the myeloma in the same way that it had in Stacy."

He says that Stacy had less than a quarter of a pound of tumor in her body at the time she underwent treatment. The patients he subsequently tried to treat on a compassionate basis had between two and six pounds of tumor in their bodies.

"That clearly is biting off more than we can chew," he says.

He used the information he gained from these patients under compassionate use to improve his clinical trial. "We're looking at people who are more like Stacy was at the time she was treated to find out whether that's the sweet spot. We don't think it was a fluke, because we've had other patients who've had quite a significant reduction in their myeloma burden—but just not to the same extent as Stacy."

Dr. Russell believes in providing dying patients access to experimental treatments outside of clinical trials. "If I see a patient who's out of options who wants to try something then my perspective is, well who am I to block that? And if I'm in a position to help them get compassionate use then I would like to do so."

However, he says, current FDA rules can make it difficult to justify taking the risk of providing experimental medicines on compassionate grounds.

"If a patient receiving an experimental therapy dies and the experimental therapy is somehow implicated in causing the death, it can derail the development of a drug," he says. "And so the entire group of patients that could benefit may either not benefit, or the benefit may be greatly delayed, because the pathway to approval is compromised."

He continues, "[In a] hypothetical situation where somebody's going to die next week, and you kind of do the Hail Mary and you give them the experimental therapy, and they die next week, then you have to be able to hand-on-heart say the drug had no part to play in this patient's death. And you can't do that. The drug may have been implicated and then FDA are all over you because they want to make sure that no one is exposed to unnecessary risk.

"So I see both sides of it," he says. If he were a manufacturer, he might not be so eager to support compassionate use, "but you know, as a physician with a patient I'm more focused on the needs of the patient who I'm seeing."

Dr. Russell knows what it is like to see someone you love denied access to an experimental treatment, because he lost a cousin to cancer who could not get access to an investigational drug he was working on.

A few years after he moved from the United Kingdom to Minnesota to take his current post at the Mayo Clinic, Dr. Russell says, "I had a cousin who was in his early fifties with a young child, he had myeloma. He'd had all available therapies and he was relapsing and looked like he'd probably die soon."

At the time, doctors at the Mayo Clinic were developing a myeloma drug called Velcade that he believed could help his cousin.

"I knew that Velcade was a good drug and we were using it in clinical trials. So I tried to get him compassionate use and they wouldn't do it. And I was just—as far as I was concerned the system was completely wrong and stupid for disallowing that. And I still would maintain that, because I think there was enough evidence on the safety efficacy profile of Velcade to justify it.

"I was very upset," he says. "It seemed like the people developing the drugs just had no real interest in sob stories, and were more concerned about the pathway to market and the profits. So I totally agree with [compassionate use] up to a point. But I can see how you do have to weigh it, depending on what stage of development the drug's at and depending on what the data available is."

Meanwhile, Stacy Erholtz has made the transition from cancer patient to patient advocate.

"This could potentially be the cure to cancer," she recently told *Medical Daily*. "If we can start treating cancer with measles, let's do it and remove all barriers in the process.

"I want people to join me in remission right now."[8]

Dr. Russell believes this treatment could become a "single shot cure for cancer."[9] He and his colleagues at the Mayo Clinic are now testing the effectiveness of the measles virus against ovarian, brain, head, and neck cancers, as well as against mesothelioma, a cancer that attacks the tissue lining the lungs, stomach, heart, and other organs.

Doctors may soon be able to harness other viruses to kill cancer as well. Dr. Russell points to research being done at Duke University using polio virus to treat glioblastoma, a deadly brain cancer.

"Polio is a virus that naturally damages the spinal cord, so it has a propensity to destroy nervous tissue," Dr. Russell says. "But what was done in this case was the virus was engineered to remove a critical component, and replace it with the identical component taken from a common cold virus. And the result was this engineered polio virus that can't any longer damage the brain or the central nervous system, but can still damage tumors that are located at that site.

"It's early stage, it's phase I," he says, "but they have had some remarkable outcomes in a small number of patients whose tumors have shrunk—quite dramatically actually—following the injection of the virus into the tumor."

The treatment was recently featured on CBS's *60 Minutes*, where a correspondent, Scott Pelley, interviewed the first person ever treated with polio virus—a twenty-year-old nursing student named Stephanie Lipscomb.

When Stephanie came to the hospital complaining of headaches in 2011, doctors took a scan and found a brain tumor the size of a tennis ball. Subsequent tests confirmed she had glioblastoma. She underwent surgery, in which doctors removed 98 percent of the tumor, followed by radiation and chemotherapy.

But a year later, her cancer was back with a vengeance. She was out of treatment options—except for one that had never been tried on a human being before. Doctors told her about the new polio treatment. They would take a needle and inject the polio virus into her brain, directly into the tumor.

When her mother heard that they wanted to inject polio into her daughter's brain, she wanted to walk out of the hospital. Stephanie was scared, but she decided to give it a try.

"I had nothing to lose, honestly," she told CBS.

So she underwent the procedure. At first, scans showed the tumor had grown after the treatment. Glioblastoma tumors are aggressive, doubling in size every two to three weeks, and Stephanie's appeared to be growing. Doctors thought the treatment wasn't working.

But it turned out that this was part of the immune reaction. As Scott Pelley reports, "Five months after her infusion, an MRI showed that the tumor hadn't been growing at all. . . . Stephanie's immune system had awakened to the cancer and gone to war."[10]

The tumor began to shrink. And after twenty-one months, it was completely gone. Today, Dr. Annick Desjardins, the physician oversee-ing her treatment, says, "She is cancer free."[11]

When they upped the dose in a subsequent patient, it caused an immune reaction that was too strong. The patient pulled out of the trial and later died. But now doctors believe they have determined the optimal dose. Of the twenty-two patients in the phase I trial, half have shown significant improvement and four are in remission.

Now Duke researchers are testing the polio vaccine against other cancers in a petri dish. "We have done this for lung cancers, breast can-cers, colorectal cancers, prostate cancers, pancreatic cancers, liver can-cers, renal cancers," said Dr. Matthias Gromeier, the Duke molecular biologist who's been working on this treatment for a quarter century.

Dr. Henry Friedman, the deputy director of Duke's brain tumor center, said, "This, to me, is the most promising therapy I've seen in my career, period."[12]

In Oregon doctors at the Providence Cancer Center are working on another potentially revolutionary glioblastoma treatment—this one using not a deadly virus but a deadly bacteria called *Listeria*.[13] *Liste-ria* attacks the brain and central nervous system. Researchers believe that by adding cancer-specific proteins to *Listeria*, they can teach the immune system to think that cancer cells are a dangerous bacterial infection and attack them.

"By putting the two together, the bacteria and the tumor, we teach the immune cells that this target is bad and needs to be destroyed," Dr. Marka Crittenden, the principal investigator, said in an article on the hospital website.[14] "This is an appealing area for immunotherapy because if we can get the immune system involved in controlling this tumor, we may be able to eliminate those other areas where micro-scopic residual tumor remains."

The study is only in phase I trials. But even if it proves safe, it will take years to make it broadly available to cancer patients. Dr. Keith

Bahjat, the director of the immune monitoring lab at Providence, says, "These studies take a significant amount of time and significant amounts of money. If money were unlimited, which it is not, we could see this push through clinical studies, and if the results are positive, have an application submitted to the FDA as an approved drug in five to six years' time."[15]

In Ohio, the *Minneapolis Star Tribune* reports, doctors at the James Cancer Hospital and Solove Research Institute are working on a vaccine "to treat pancreatic cancer using Reolysin, a proprietary variant of the virus that causes the common cold."[16] The principal investigator, Dr. Tanios Bekaii-Saab, told the paper "he expects one of these virus 'platforms' is likely to become standard treatment for a cancer such as myeloma or pancreatic cancer within three to four years."

In the United Kingdom researchers have developed a vaccine to treat melanoma using the herpes simplex virus. "The virus was obtained from the cold sore of a patient who worked at the company," Dr. Russell of the Mayo Clinic says. "It was grown on cultured cells. It was engineered by removing a couple of the viral genes that make it capable of causing damage. . . . And an additional gene was added in to enhance its ability to stimulate the immune system."

The British researchers used it on patients who, Dr. Russell says, "had melanoma that had spread all over their skin. And what they would do with the virus is just inject one site repeatedly every two weeks with virus. And what happened in proportion to the patients was that the melanoma everywhere resolved. And so it was a local injection of the virus. It spread locally; it didn't spread via the bloodstream to other sites, so there was destruction of the melanoma cells at the injection site and then there was this dramatic immune activation and immune mediated destruction of the melanoma at other sites."

The vaccine recently completed a phase III trial with about 430 patients, and it had a "durable response"—meaning the tumor goes away and does not return—in about 16 percent of melanoma patients, compared with 2 percent in a control group. The drug, called T-VEC, was bought by Amgen, which is seeking FDA approval for it.

Perhaps one of the most amazing developments in viral therapy is taking place at Children's Hospital in Philadelphia, where doctors are harnessing the power of one of the worst killers in the history of viruses—HIV, the virus that causes AIDS—to cure leukemia.

In this revolutionary treatment, doctors don't inject the virus into a tumor or even infuse a genetically altered virus into the bloodstream.

They genetically engineer the patient's *own blood* to kill cancer.

In cancers such as acute lymphoblastic leukemia (ALL), certain cells in the blood called B-cells become cancerous. Normally, T-cells—special white blood cells that are the predators in the body's immune system—would hunt down the cancer and kill it. But in ALL, the B-cells have developed a cloaking mechanism that allows them to fly under the radar of the killer T-cells.

In T-cell immunotherapy, doctors draw blood from the patients and separate out T-cells. They then use a disabled form of the HIV virus (which knows how to infect T-cells) to insert a special gene that reprograms the T-cells to recognize and attack the cancerous B-cells. The genetically altered T-cells are then infused back into the patient's body, where they go to war with the cancer.

"The virus has been engineered so that it can't cause disease anymore," says Dr. Carl June, the oncologist at the University of Pennsylvania who pioneered the technique. "But it still retains the ability to reprogram the immune system so that it will now attack cancer cells. We call those modified immune cells 'serial killer' cells. Each infused cell can kill more than a thousand different tumor cells."[17]

In April 2012 a seven-year-old girl named Emily Whitehead became the first child ever to undergo T-cell immunotherapy treatment. Two years earlier, when Emily was just five years old, she was diagnosed with ALL. About 90 percent of children under fifteen respond to a special combination of chemotherapy drugs first pioneered in the 1960s by

Dr. Emil Freireich, a professor at MD Anderson Cancer Center.[18] But Emily was among the minority of patients in whom it did not work. She underwent two rounds of chemotherapy, but relapsed each time.

"We spent two years in the hospital," says Tom Whitehead, Emily's father.

She was running out of options, and the Whiteheads began looking into experimental therapies. They reached out to Children's Hospital, where doctors told them about a phase I trial for the new T-cell therapy. Doctors explained why they were hopeful for the treatment, and that it had already worked in several adults. But they also told the Whiteheads that a phase I trial was intended not to cure the patient, but rather to determine the safety and optimal dose of the drug.

At first the Whiteheads were not sure. "My wife's in research at Penn State so she looked into it, and she just said we're not ready to just try a trial to find out what dose will work for future patients, we need something that will help Emily," Tom says.

But then Emily started declining rapidly. Doctors said her major organs could fail within days. With their beloved daughter slipping away, they decided to try the experimental therapy.

Doctors removed Emily's blood, reengineered her T-cells, and then infused them back into her body. The adults who had undergone the procedure had experienced mild flu-like symptoms, but Emily became violently ill. She developed chills and then a raging fever that spiked to 105. Her blood pressure plummeted, her lungs flooded, and she was rushed to the pediatric intensive care unit, where she ended up on a ventilator.

"At one point they told me that there's a one in a thousand chance Emily would survive the night," Tom says, "and that was pretty tough to hear."

With Emily at death's door, her doctors figured out that the level of an immune protein called IL-6 had become elevated as a result of the T-cells growing in her body. Then Dr. June hit on an idea: his daughter was taking a medication for juvenile rheumatoid arthritis that is known to turn off production of that same protein. He gave it to Emily. It worked. Emily stabilized. Her fever broke, and her T-cells went to work fighting the cancer.

A week later, on her birthday, she woke up. And twenty-eight days after her treatment, doctors conducted a bone-marrow examination to look for cancer. They could not find any. None. Zero. They could not believe it. Doctors tried the test again and came up with the same result. Her cancer was completely gone.

"It was like the calm after the storm," Dr. June says. "The clouds went away and she woke up and there was no leukemia. When that child survived, it was of course an amazing event."[19]

As of May 10, 2015, she's been in remission for three years. The genetically altered T-cells are still in her body, protecting her against a recurrence of the cancer.

Since Emily underwent her treatment, *Forbes* reports, thirty people (twenty-five other children and five adults) have undergone the same treatment. Of those, twenty-seven have had a full remission.[20]

T-cell immunotherapy is being backed by the pharmaceutical giant Novartis. It is a risky investment that breaks the traditional mold of "blockbuster" drugs that can be mass-produced for multiple patients. The vaccine is unlike other cancer treatments—even cutting-edge viral therapies—because the company cannot mass-produce it. Each dose must be custom-made using the patient's own blood. It is truly personalized medicine.

Novartis CEO Joseph Jimenez told *Forbes*, "I've told the team that resources are not an issue. Speed is the issue. I want to hear what it takes to run this Phase III trial and get this to market. You're talking about patients who are about to die. The pain of having to turn patients away is such that we are going as fast as we can and not letting resources get in the way."[21]

Novartis is to be commended for investing in this technology. But Jimenez's statement raises a question: if resources are not an issue, why does Novartis have to turn patients away? It is one thing for a tiny biotech like Sarepta—which literally has no cash to produce a drug outside of clinical trials—to say that it cannot provide its drug under compassionate use.

But why can't a company like Novartis provide it?

I asked Novartis how many patients had been turned away. A Novartis spokesman, Scott Young, did not give a specific answer, but said, "Decisions regarding treatment have been based on strictly defined eligibility criteria agreed with the FDA."

The fact is, for Emily Whitehead, Stephanie Lipscomb, and Stacy Erholtz, the experimental treatment came just in time. But for many other desperately ill Americans, the chance to save their lives never comes. The American Cancer Society estimates that about 1,450 Americans will die of acute lymphoblastic leukemia, the cancer Emily beat, in 2015.[22] Another thirteen thousand will die of glioblastoma, the cancer that afflicted Stephanie,[23] while some eleven thousand will die of multiple myeloma, the cancer that nearly killed Stacy.[24]

These dying Americans don't have access to promising new therapies. And while there is no guarantee such therapies would save them, most dying patients are not looking for a guarantee—they just want a fighting chance. And at the current pace of drug approvals—even under the FDA's painfully slow accelerated approval process—most of these treatments will not be available to patients for many years.

One person who says that this needs to change is Dr. Freireich, the doctor who discovered the standard treatment for Emily's cancer— childhood ALL—five decades ago. He believes patients with terminal diagnoses should not have to wait for the government to approve next-generation treatments. "The FDA is preventing . . . physicians from making decisions about treatment, patients making decisions about their own healthcare. It's doing everything that we as a country believe is wrong. Fundamentally wrong," he says. "When a patient has a terminal illness and is not eligible to participate in a drug-testing program that is FDA-approved, they should have access to that drug if their physician and they want to take that risk."[25]

Another person who agrees is Dr. John Bell, an award-winning scientist at the Center for Innovative Cancer Research at Ottawa Hospital Research Institute in Canada.[26] Dr. Bell is considered one of the pioneers of modern oncolytic viral therapy. He was the first scientist to show that vaccinia viruses, used in smallpox vaccine, could be delivered intravenously to infect and kill cancer tumors without harming normal tissue in patients.[27]

He is also a big advocate for expanding access to experimental therapies.

"I think it's absolutely critical," he says. "If we have therapies that work, there's no reason not to treat people with those."

Like most doctors who are working on the cutting edge of cancer research, Dr. Bell gets inundated with requests from desperate patients. "I get phone calls every day," he says, "and I have to say, 'Sorry, I can't offer you anything.'

"There's a huge need in society for the solution to this problem," he says. "I think there should be more access to these experimental therapeutics. So we need to expand access to these and allow us to give more experimentation in combinations to people who really want to have a shot at it, rather than just have palliative care that's really only going to potentially maybe reduce pain—maybe not—and maybe actually just make their life more unpleasant."

He says viral therapies are safe. The fact is, we give people viruses all the time, without FDA testing. When kids go to get a flu vaccine, they're getting flu virus. And when kids get measles vaccine, they're getting measles virus. So we inject viruses into people every day. "That's why we're not worried about safety because we have a tremendous safety profile from the last two hundred years of vaccinations."

Not only are viral therapies safe; they are far milder on cancer patients than most approved treatments. "These therapies are much more benign then chemo and radiation therapy by a long stretch and that's good," he says. "So even if they were only as effective as chemotherapy, the fact that they're much less toxic is a good thing.

"I don't want to say chemotherapy is horrible," he adds. "We actually have some studies showing that some kinds of chemotherapy in combination with viruses actually do much better." But, he says, "Our current chemo and radiation therapies are not curing people with metastatic disease, which is a lot of people. So since we're not curing them anyhow, why not give them the option [to try investigational treatments]?"

No treatment is without risk, he says, but "lots of people die every day from chemotherapy. So let's just get over ourselves here and say this isn't working, we're paying a lot of money for it, we're putting people in the hospital with these treatments; we should really start to try to move forward faster.

"I think it's unethical in my opinion—it's unethical to withhold these treatments if there's a potential there. It's unethical to treat people with things we know are not going to cure them and that could make them very, very sick," he says.

There is no guarantee that patients will have the same miraculous response as Stacy Erholtz, Emily Whitehead, and Stephanie Lipscomb. But, Dr. Bell says, "a 16 percent [chance] is better than zero, and maybe 1 percent is better than zero and maybe a small percentage is better if you have a therapy that doesn't basically debilitate you."

One of the criticisms of Right to Try is that it will drive patients into the arms of charlatans. But Dr. Bell says that it is the lack of access to promising therapies with real science behind them that is driving people to quacks.

"In cancer there's a lot of really bad people who exploit people's desperation. There's a guy in Ottawa who calls himself 'Dr. Hope' who basically gets people to give him money and he promises them good outcomes with really no good basis in science or therapies that make any sense at all."

He says of the FDA, "In fairness, they're trying to keep people from being exploited." But he adds that "the problem is they're actually not [protecting people]. We over-engineer our regulatory system to try to keep [bad] people from benefitting. And we don't stop them. They still carry on. And it just makes it harder for people like myself, who are willing to do science the right way, to get going forward. It's just bizarre, and it's also bad for the patients."

Tom Whitehead, Emily's father, agrees. Before Emily got access to an experimental treatment, when it seemed they were out of options, Tom says they thought about traveling abroad. "I can tell you that was a consideration of ours. There were different times when we thought it's possible we might have to go overseas. Because doctors would tell us, 'Hey, there's this thing in Germany . . . that's not approved here yet.'

"I've seen families that went to Mexico, where they told them they'll heat their body up to a certain temperature and different things. When you're desperate, you're going to try something if you can't get anything here, I guarantee it.

"As a parent," he says, "you would do anything to save your child."

Dr. Bell supports Right to Try laws. "It's a great idea," he says. "Our societies are too paternalistic. We think we know better than the patient, what they really want.

"Society wants this and I don't know why we're sort of stuck in this quagmire."

He believes we are at the cusp of unprecedented breakthroughs in cancer treatment. "I've been doing this for a long time, about thirty years in this field, and I've never seen the developments like we've seen in the last five years," he says.

# 5.

# Inside Man

*How One Biotech CEO Came to Champion Right to Try*

———

When the Goldwater Institute first launched Right to Try, it was immediately embraced by doctors, patients, and legislators across the country. But at first, no one in the pharmaceutical or biotechnology industries stepped forward to openly support the idea . . . until, that is, one courageous CEO of a cutting-edge biotech firm came out publicly and declared: Yes, dying Americans do have the Right to Try.

"THAT'S MY SON'S BRAIN tumor."

Richard Garr points to a shelf in his office. Among the books, awards, mementos, and scientific models sits a large misshapen piece of plastic. He picks it up and holds it in his hand.

It is the size of a grapefruit.

"They make a mold of it with computers," Garr says. "He had a tumor when he was very small, when he was four years old."

Twenty-three years ago, Garr's son Matthew began complaining about disabling pain in his neck. The pain came and went, and doctors never thought it was anything serious. Then one day, during a routine eye exam, his optician looked into the back of Matthew's eyes and saw signs of enormous pressure. He said it probably was nothing, but suggested that Matthew should have an MRI done.

"We sort of knew immediately it wasn't 'nothing,'" Garr says. And indeed, the MRI showed a massive tumor in Matthew's brain.

Within a week, he was on the operating table at National Children's Medical Center in Washington. The surgery took eighteen hours. The tumor had wrapped itself around Matthew's brain stem, and removing it was incredibly complicated. Thankfully, Dr. Dennis Johnson, one of the leading neurosurgeons in the country, was able to perform the surgery.

"We were fortunate that Dr. Johnson was available," Garr says. "There are very few guys even in that elite universe who could do what he did, get it all out without killing him. We are more blessed than you can imagine."

After Matthew's surgery, he lay in a coma for several weeks. When he finally recovered and was able to return to school, he had to start kindergarten a year late.

That delay would end up saving Ted Harada's life . . . and change the course of medical history.

When Matthew finally began classes at the McLean School in Potomac, Maryland, he became best friends with a classmate named Arthur Johe. The two boys spent a lot of time together outside school, and Richard Garr became friends with Arthur's dad, Karl. When Richard told Karl about Matthew's surgery, Karl's response shocked him:

"Well, someday we'll be able to fix that."

Karl Johe, it turned out, was a scientist at the National Institutes of Health (NIH). And not just any scientist. Johe had discovered neural stem cells, which can grow to become brain or spinal cord cells. The two men bonded over their shared interest in brain science.

Garr, who was then a successful real estate attorney, was looking for something he could do to help his son and others like him. "Every parent of every child who faces a life-threatening illness looks for a way to help," Garr says. "Usually you end up helping to raise money for charity, or getting involved with the brain tumor society or something like that. And Lisa, my wife, and I, we did all those things."

But Garr felt a growing passion to do more.

Meanwhile, Johe was feeling a growing frustration with the NIH and the politics of obtaining research grants. So in 1997 the two men decided to go into business together.

"We ended up starting a company, which is very unusual in the life sciences," Garr says. "You see it in high tech—two guys in a garage. You don't see that in biology. But we did it."

Soon Neuralstem was born. And at this writing, eighteen years later, Garr is among the longest-serving CEOs in the stem-cell industry.

As we have seen at the start of this book, their work in the ensuing decades produced a modern-day medical miracle, when Ted Harada became the first person in recorded medical history to see his ALS symptoms reversed. "Our goal," Garr says, "is to try and turn ALS into a chronic manageable disease as opposed to a fatal disease."

But Neuralstem's technology has applications far beyond treatment of ALS. The company is also targeting a host of other major central nervous system conditions.

"We are also treating ischemic stroke, actually in China; those are direct injections in the brain," Garr says. "And we have two spinal cord injury trials. One that started in UC San Diego which is for chronic spinal cord injury . . . where there is no sensory or motor function below the injury. Then we're setting up an acute spinal cord injury trial in Seoul, which is right after the accident."

Another area in which neural stem cells show promise is as a platform for treating depression, a deadly disease that leads to tens of thousands of suicides a year in the United States.[1] In the late 1990s,

Neuralstem won a contract to work on the Pentagon's "War Fighter of the Future" project. "[They] came to us and said, 'We'd like you to put your cells in dishes and screen against them to find a new class of drugs that will cognitively enhance the soldiers,'" Garr says.

The drug they developed, which is now in clinical trials, is a small molecule pill that may stimulate the brain's capacity to generate new neurons. If it works, it has the potential to treat central nervous system conditions such as major depressive disorder (MDD), traumatic brain injury, cognitive deficit and schizophrenia, and post-traumatic stress disorder (PTSD).[2]

Garr explains how it works: "So inside your head you're pretty much hardwired. But there's an area of your brain called the hippocampus, which is sort of like your processing center where all your thinking and a lot of your emotions are seated.

"And your hippocampus actually has a little bit of a reservoir of neural stem cells—not the hardwired, fully adaptive neurons and nuclei, but their precursor cells," Garr says. "And through life they sort of replenish the hippocampus with new synaptic contacts. You have more of them when you are young, and fewer of them when you're old, and so maybe that's why it's easier to learn a language and things . . . when you're young.

"Well, we can grow those precursor cells in dishes," Garr says. "That's what our technology is. It's growing stem cells."

Neuralstem just completed a phase Ib trial of the pill. According to Garr, "We released the data last summer. The top guy in the field at Harvard did our trial, released the data, and it showed that in fact we reduced depression and the cognitive deficit in the depressed patients in a clinically meaningful way. Statistically significant and clinically meaningful. And so we're going into a phase II now to treat depression and we expect to start a trial to treat the cognitive deficit in schizophrenia."

Asked by an interviewer recently if the pill could one day reverse some of the effects of aging, Dr. Johe said, "Yes, there's no question that degeneration of the hippocampus and other parts of the brain is part of the aging process. As we now take many different food supplements to counter or slow that aging process, I see this as a potential 'vitamin for the brain' to slow down or counter that aging process in our mental capacity."[3]

One of the most dreaded neurological diseases affecting aging Americans is Alzheimer's. At the University of Michigan, Dr. Eva Feldman—the doctor who pioneered the neural-stem-cell treatment that reversed Ted Harada's ALS symptoms—is now developing stem-cell surgery that might one day reverse the symptoms of Alzheimer's.

The *Detroit News* reports that Dr. Feldman recently completed pre-clinical trials that showed that neural stem cells had a remarkable impact on mice engineered with the gene that causes Alzheimer's.[4] In the study, Dr. Feldman injected one group of mice with neural stem cells into their hippocampus, while a second group was injected with saline solution. She then evaluated the two groups by giving them memory tests.

"Those animals [who got the neural stem cells] retained their ability to think, as a mouse does, to recognize objects so they looked just like an animal that doesn't have Alzheimer's disease," she told the paper. "It's really remarkable."

"When you work in science, you do as many experiments that don't work as that do," Dr. Feldman said. "When you get something that works so beautifully (like this experiment), you can quickly see its translational potential. I am looking at a mouse but someday I could be looking at a man. As a clinician scientist, those are the moments you live for."

She's still a long way away from human testing. But the results hold great promise for a fatal disease that is estimated to affect as many as five million Americans age sixty-five and older.

I first learned about Garr and Neuralstem during the fight to pass Arizona's Right to Try law. One day I was scanning stories about Right to Try when a blog post Garr wrote on Neuralstem's company website caught my eye.[5]

"The 'Right to Try' bill is making its way through the (now infamous) Arizona State Legislature," Garr wrote. "The Arizona State Legislature is the incubator of some of the worst laws in the history of bad laws, embodying obviously hateful and penal opposition to all manner of group."

Oh boy, I thought, here we go.

But then came the surprise twist:

"I suspect that this bill may resonate broadly both in and outside of Arizona," he wrote.

Huh? I checked his bio again. This was coming from the CEO of a biotech company?

Quoting the reggae legend Bob Marley ("Every man gotta right to decide his own destiny") Garr continued:

The basic premise of the Bill is that patients with fatal and incurable diseases should be able to choose for themselves whether or not to try an experimental drug. The Bill's authors state that they should not be constrained by the FDA's approval process. . . .

The Bill was drafted by the libertarian leaning Goldwater Institute, and is based on the premise that the FDA's approval process denies citizens the right to choose their own medical path. The Bill stipulates that it only applies to fatal diseases, and only to medicines that have passed a FDA Phase I safety trial, and further to medicines that are currently in (at least) a FDA Phase II trial; so there is some effort to restrict the scope of this program to drugs that have had a good level of FDA scrutiny. There must still be a licensed medical doctor involved to prescribe the investigational drug; and the law states that companies cannot be forced to provide the drug if they so choose. Finally, there is language that looks to allow for companies to charge for these treatments. The provision is vague but seems to reference cost reimbursement language.

At Neuralstem we are keeping a sharp eye on this legislation.

As we move into the final stretch of transplantations for our Phase II therapy for ALS . . . we are keenly aware of all of the patients who cannot be included in the trial; both because of the small number of patients in the trial, and also because of the exclusive nature of inclusion/exclusion criteria the trial is built around. And as we begin to design the next trial, a trial which we hope will lead to approval by the FDA, we are thinking more and more about ways to broaden access to our cells.

We support the intent of this bill. One does not have to be a fire breathing libertarian to wish that cutting edge technology could get to its intended recipients sooner and with less red tape. . . . Right to Try is a good idea with lots of flaws; but a good idea nonetheless, and an idea worth supporting and pursuing.

I immediately picked up the phone and called him.

He seemed surprised to hear from me. "My personal politics are 180 degrees from Goldwater," he said. "I'm your typical knee-jerk Democrat, born and raised in Washington, lifelong liberal."

We began discussing Right to Try. He told me that "from the land of the worst ideas ever, this is not such a bad idea. It has flaws, but there are ways this could really help the ALS community in particular." I candidly asked him why he was so willing to support the Right to Try when most CEOs were taking the "don't rock the boat" approach, not wanting to get crosswise with the FDA. He said that even if his company's ALS treatment proved successful, by the time it reached the market, all his patients outside the few in the clinical trials would be dead. Garr would spend hours at night emailing and talking with patients desperate to get into his ongoing trials, and he was powerless to help. He wanted to get those patients, and other terminal patients, faster access to promising new treatments.

So I asked him to work with me and help us fix the flaws. He agreed.

Weeks later, Garr and I published an article in *USA Today* asking the FDA and legislators to support the Right to Try. Today Garr speaks out for Right to Try at biotech industry meetings and conferences on rare diseases.

When he started making the case for Right to Try, he says, "The industry push-back shocked me.

"They would say all these terrible things like, 'Well, who's going to pay for it? How are you going to control the proper consent to the patients? How do you know they're not being scammed?' And my answer was: Well, yeah, those are all real questions. And by the way it's going to pass anyway, and they're going to get dumped in your lap. So rather than fight it and say this is a horrible idea and wring your hands, you should get inside and get behind it and make sure that it addresses all these questions. They're all legitimate questions."

He says he is slowly making progress.

"They're coming around to the point where they'll actually talk to me," he says.

He is sympathetic to the concerns the critics raise. "My view is that there are real issues that have to be resolved. Who is going to pay for this? Are the insurance companies going to reimburse for this? If they don't, does this mean only rich people are going to be able to access Right to Try?"

But, he says, "there are people in our industry who spend all day, every day, figuring out who pays for what and why. So this isn't peace in the Middle East, right? These are tough questions, but there are people who do that all the time. You may not like their answers, but don't tell me there's no way to get to that answer, right?"

He says his approach is to tell his colleagues, "Let me explain why you should support it—not why I'm right and you're wrong—why *you* should support it. What we're telling industry is, look, you're going to be under pressure to provide this anyway. You don't want to be on TV and some woman holding her child saying, 'They wouldn't give me the emergency drugs, my child's going to die.'"

It is better for industry to support Right to Try and help solve the very real challenges, he says, than to be standing outside opposing it while a large, grassroots political movement demanding access grows across the country.

He says the logistics can be solved. As evidence, he points out that "nobody had any problem getting around all the issues with Ebola."

In July 2014, when the American medical missionary Dr. Kent Brantly was caring for Ebola patients in Liberia and contracted the deadly disease, he was given an experimental antiviral drug called ZMapp, which was produced by the San Diego–based Mapp Biopharmaceutical. It had undergone no human clinical trials or safety tests before it was given to Dr. Brantly. Indeed, it had never been tried on human beings before. When the Ebola outbreak happened, the *New York Times* reported, Mapp had just been "gearing up to start the larger animal toxicity studies typically needed before testing it in humans, with an eye on doing the first human safety studies in healthy volunteers" in 2015.[6]

In all, at least six people are known to have received ZMapp, according to the World Health Organization. Two have recovered, three have shown improvement, and one has died.

According to the *Washington Post*, the FDA allowed the makers of ZMapp and two other experimental Ebola drugs "permission to use the unapproved medications on humans, even though their safety and effectiveness against Ebola has not been proven."[7] Indeed, the Obama administration has asked Congress for $58 million to ramp up production and testing of ZMapp and to speed the development of two other experimental treatments.

The assistant general director of the World Health Organization, Marie-Paule Kieny, praised the FDA for its willingness to clear safety and bureaucratic hurdles so quickly, calling the speed of action "absolutely unprecedented.

"We have to change the sense that there is no hope," she said.[8]

For Jenn McNary—the mom we met in chapter 1 whose son can't

get access to a promising Duchenne drug—watching the FDA clear bureaucratic red tape to allow dying patients to try untested, experimental treatments was bittersweet.

"I read about Ebola and how drug companies are able to just sort of take this drug wherever because it is an emergency," she says. "Duchenne is also an emergency. Kids die from this disease every day. It is the most common lethal genetic disorder in children."

How could the FDA throw out the rule book to permit the use of a treatment for Ebola that has not been proved safe or effective, while at the same time denying Jenn's son, Austin, access to a drug that has been shown to be safe and effective in his own brother? How can the FDA permit the use of an Ebola drug that has never even been tested on a human being while denying cancer patients access to medicines that have passed phase I, phase II, and sometimes phase III FDA testing?

Garr says the answer is simple: Ebola is contagious.

"Duchenne disease is not contagious. ALS is not contagious. Cancer is not contagious. So society has answered that question. We're willing to waive all these issues if it's contagious and it can affect me. We're not willing to waive all these issues without a big fight if it's not. I mean, that's where I see it sitting right now."

When Ebola arrived in America, Garr says, "nobody hesitated two seconds. All these other questions went out the window with Ebola immediately. Pull everybody off of everything, we'll figure out how you get paid later . . . give it to them, give it to them, give it to them.

"In my mind, the Ebola situation should have just evaporated any arguments, all the other arguments that people had against [Right to Try]," he says.

While there are legitimate issues that need to be resolved when it comes to implementing Right to Try, many objections raised by critics are based on a misunderstanding of what the law does and does not do. For example, there is a perception that Right to Try laws cut the FDA out of the picture. One of the nation's leading cancer specialists actually said in an interview for this book, "Right to Try is 'I'm dying of cancer, there's this new drug that's been given to seven dogs, three chimpanzees, and one human being, and I'm saying I demand that drug today.'"

That is not what Right to Try is.

Quite the opposite, as Garr explained in a recent blog post: "The FDA is an indispensable party in this process. Indeed the [Right to Try] bill relies heavily on their expertise and diligence. That is why the bill only applies to fatal diseases, and only to drugs or therapies that have passed an FDA-approved safety trial, and are still actively being developed under the FDA umbrella in further trials.

"The FDA is not the enemy," Garr says.[9]

The problem is that the existing emergency structures from the FDA are not adequate to meet the rising demand for access to emerging drugs. That's because compassionate use is designed for small numbers of people who are seeking access to later-stage AIDS and cancer drugs for which there have been big trials but the drug is still a few years away from approval. It is not designed for broad access by large numbers of patients to early-stage innovative technology that is showing promise in small trials and could make a difference for patients with an unmet need.

The Right to Try movement is demanding that kind of access to investigational drugs on a much broader scale—and the current system is not designed to accommodate that demand.

Garr points out that Right to Try presents different challenges to small and large companies. Many small companies can't afford to accommodate compassionate use requests. "If you're Glaxo or Merck, it doesn't cost you anything to manufacture a thousand pills," Garr says. "But most of these innovative drugs are coming out of . . . small biotechs."

He is right. As we saw earlier in the case of Sarepta and its Duchenne drug, eteplirsen, small companies don't always have the resources to produce enough drugs or to cover their costs for patients to get compassionate use.

He says the challenge for the big pharmaceutical companies—those who *can* afford it—is that they are afraid that providing access to experimental treatments, even under the existing FDA-approved compassionate use system, will put their investments at risk.

"The way the FDA works is if you put your drug in somebody—whether it's approved or not—and something bad happens, you have to tell the FDA," Garr says. "If that person dies, the FDA could stop their trial."

For a major new drug, that could cost the company millions and delay getting the drug to market.

"So that's where big pharma, that's the real push-back you get from the people who can afford to do this," he says.

To make Right to Try work on a large scale, companies need some guarantee that if they offer an experimental treatment to someone who does not meet the criteria of a clinical trial—because the patient has complications or is in a late stage and at high risk of dying—the FDA is not going to stop their trial if that high-risk patient dies.

By contrast, he says, "if you can protect them against the negative [of] having it affect their clinical trials, if you can protect them, then there's nothing but upside for them to treat these higher-risk patients, because if something goes wrong they're not going to lose their clinical trial, they're not going to get liability, but the payoff is somebody with a late stage or something is cured, the publicity and everything that comes with it is dramatic."

Others have raised concerns that Right to Try laws will push terminal patients into the arms of quacks with unproven treatments who prey on the desperation of dying Americans. But Ted Harada—the ALS survivor whose symptoms were reversed thanks to Garr and Johe's technology—says the opposite is true.

"The FDA is pushing us to the snake-oil salesmen," Ted says. "Because someone dying is going to try anything—*anything*. People don't want to die without hope. The FDA pushes them into trying riskier things."

Today, the world outside the United States is filled with nefarious characters taking advantage of the sick and dying, promising cures for everything from brain tumors to Alzheimer's. People are holding bake sales and fund-raisers to send their children to Colombia, Mexico, and other countries for false cures.

A few years ago, the *Wall Street Journal* reported: "Some patients with fatal Lou Gehrig's disease, frustrated by the slow pace of clinical drug trials or unable to qualify, are trying to brew their own version of an experimental compound at home and testing it on themselves."[10]

Such actions show how desperate the ALS community is, Ted says.

Right to Try laws actually direct people away from false cures like these by giving them access to treatments at home that have real science behind them. Before a drug can even begin a phase I trial and be put into a human being, a company must spend millions of dollars and show the FDA reams of data from laboratory testing and animal studies. So once a drug completes phase I trials, it has tens of millions of research dollars behind it. Those that complete phase II trials and move into phase III have even more scientific data behind them and an even better chance of eventual success. These treatments are not guaranteed to work. But unlike quack treatments that patients will find abroad, they have a real *chance* of working.

This is why critics are wrong when they say Right to Try gives patients false hope. Terminal patients who have exhausted all the FDA-approved treatments have *no hope*. Right to Try does not promise them a cure; it offers them a *chance*. It gives terminal patients real hope by granting access to promising investigational treatments. Denying them that hope—telling them to go home and die when there is still a chance, even a remote chance, to save their lives—is flat-out cruel.

There are solutions to all the challenges we face, Garr says, but we are not going to find those solutions without the forcing mechanism of Right to Try laws. "Right to Try provides a scaffold where you could build the structure to answer all these questions," Garr says. "And they're not going to get answered hypothetically. The insurance companies are not going to say, 'Okay, we'll reimburse for this' until it's put to them.

"So yes, all of these things have to be addressed," Garr says. "But again, informed consent, reimbursement, all these things are addressed by this industry all day every day for really tough questions."

Garr's point is that none of these are arguments against the Right to Try. They are challenges to overcome in *implementing* the Right to Try. We need to solve them. But we cannot allow them to become excuses for inaction.

I believe that most Americans understand this, and that this is why the Right to Try movement is sweeping the country.

# 6.

# We Are the 99 Percent

*How Right to Try Has Taken America by Storm*

---

The first Right to Try law passed in May 2014. In a little over a year since then, Right to Try has passed in twenty-four states and counting.

That is a legislative land-speed record.

And it is only a matter of time before it is the law of the land in all fifty states.

Why has Right to Try taken the country by storm? Simple: almost everywhere it has passed, courageous Americans fighting terminal illnesses have stepped forward to fight for it. These patients and their families have testified before state legislatures, lobbied their elected leaders, and shared their stories with the media—asking their fellow citizens to stand with them in the fight to save their lives.

These stories have captured the imaginations of legislators of both parties and inspired millions to rally around the terminally ill. Some of their stories have had happy endings. Others have ended tragically. In others, the final chapters are still being written.

These Americans moved hearts—and votes—in support of the principle that every American has a fundamental right to try to save his or her own life.

Let's meet some of the heroes of the Right to Try movement—starting with one who is just five years old.

## INDIANA

Like most little boys his age, Jordan McLinn wanted to be a fireman.

Unlike most little boys his age, Jordan actually got his wish—and then rallied his fellow firefighters to pass a new Indiana law that will help save lives.

On January 17, 2013, when Jordan was three, a routine visit to the pediatrician turned into a nightmare: he was diagnosed with muscular dystrophy.

But doctors did not know which kind of muscular dystrophy he had—Becker, a chronic but survivable form of the disease; or Duchenne, which is fatal. So they told Jordan's mom, Laura, to bring him to the lab on Monday to leave the blood sample that would confirm which kind it was.

"They said it would take three weeks to get that test back," Laura says. "I remember that I fasted [from] all food for almost the full three weeks and prayed so hard that it would not come back as Duchenne. It was the hardest three weeks of my life. It was like we were in mourning but trying to create hope at the same time."

Three weeks later the news finally came: Jordan had Duchenne.

"I will never forget the day I got the call," she says. "We pretty much felt like our world had come to an end." Like other Duchenne moms we have met, Laura was told that there was nothing she could do to help her son.

She was devastated.

One morning after his diagnosis, Laura was making breakfast for her family and watching the *Today* show when she saw a story that riveted her.[1] The reporter told the story of Jenn McNary and her struggle to save her sons, Max and Austin.

"Each day brings Jenn McNary another dose of hope and heartache as she watches one son get healthier while the other becomes sicker," the *Today* show correspondent said.

The correspondent interviewed Dr. Jerry Mendell, the principal investigator in Max's clinical trial. He explained how eteplirsen allowed children with Duchenne to "skip" a broken exon in their genetic code and start producing dystrophin—the protein their muscles need to avoid breaking down and maintain their function.

"Everything I can tell indicates that this is a winner," Mendell told the *Today* show "It's a game changer."

Laura was mesmerized. Could this be the cure for Jordan?

She immediately Googled Dr. Mendell. "I didn't really even know anything about exon skipping but I sent him an email and told him about Jordan. I asked him if Jordan could benefit from exon skipping and would he be willing to see Jordan," Laura says. "He emailed me back in the middle of the night, which was awesome, and told me that Jordan could be a candidate for skipping exon 53 and that that drug was coming up through the pipeline. He invited Jordan to come and be his patient."

It was the first good news Laura had gotten in months.

She took Jordan to Columbus to see Dr. Mendell. "We've had this hope that Jordan would get into the clinical trial for skipping exon 53 because they keep saying it's coming up, coming up. Well, when I talked to Sarepta a month or two ago, I called them and they said they are still on track with starting a clinical trial this summer, but you have to be seven to get in it, and Jordan will be six in May."

Just like Mindy Leffler's son, Aidan, Jordan was too healthy to be admitted into the study.

"Obviously we were heartbroken because we'd had so much hope that he would make it into this trial," Laura says.

While she kept working to save Jordan's life, Laura also focused on helping Jordan make the most of the life he had left. He was obsessed with becoming a fireman, so Laura hit on an idea she thought would bring joy to Jordan and help raise awareness for Duchenne.

She would try to get Jordan a "job" helping out at the local fire station.

"I put together a little résumé for my son to get a job as a firefighter," Laura says. "It's got a cute little picture of him in some fire gear."

The résumé read:

Jordan Joseph Nelson McLinn, Age 5

Date of Birth 5/15/09

Objective: To obtain a job at the fire station helping the firefighters.

Qualifications: I am strong. I love God. I love helping people. I am super smart.

Challenges: I have Duchenne Muscular Dystrophy. Science says within 3 to 7 years I will be in a wheelchair and within 15 years I will most likely be living in heaven because all my muscles will be deteriorated. We don't really believe that though.

Skills: Taking Care of Dogs, Cleaning, Building Things, Playing with Cars & Trucks, Dancing, Cooking, Making People Smile.

At the bottom, Laura added:

Jordan says he wants to be a firefighter when he grows up. He was given a fatal diagnosis of DMD last year. It would be awesome if there is anything he can do maybe once a week for a short time to help out at the fire station. We are pretty flexible with days/times. He is an awesome little boy, happy and full of life! Please let me know if I can bring him in for an, "interview." Thank you for your consideration.

Laura crossed her fingers, and sent the résumé to Ernest Malone, chief of the Indianapolis Fire Department.

Afterward, just for fun, she posted Jordan's résumé on her Facebook page with a message that said, "Hey, wish us luck."

It went viral.

"The next thing I know, within hours Jordan was getting job offers from New York City, Las Vegas, Alabama, Michigan," she says.

Firefighters from all over the country were reaching out to help the little boy.

Right before Christmas, Jordan had two job "interviews." One was with the firehouse at Bargersville, a small town south of Indianapolis, and another with IFD Station 13 in downtown Indianapolis.

On Christmas Eve, Jordan came to Ladder 13, and had a tour of the firehouse. He got to climb into the driver's seat of the ambulance and fire trucks, turn on the lights and sirens, and even take a slide down the fire pole. The fire department chaplain gave him a copy of the firefighters' Bible.[2]

Then Jordan sat down for his interview with Captain Tim Robinson. He was the first candidate Captain Robinson had ever interviewed who had arrived clutching a big brown teddy bear.

"Do you think you could get up every morning and help us clean the firehouse?" Captain Robinson asked him.

"Yeah," Jordan said. He asked if maybe they could call to wake him up.

"We can do that," Captain Robinson said.

"I think it went well," the captain told Jordan's mom when the interview was done, as she wiped back tears from watching her son so happy.

On Christmas, Santa delivered some good news.

"He wakes up on Christmas morning and had two letters in his stocking with job offers," Laura says. One was from Bargersville, the other from the Indianapolis Fire Department.

The letter from the IFD read:

*Dear Jordan McLinn,*

*Congratulations! You have been selected to be an honorary Firefighter for the Indianapolis Fire Department. At this time you are being given a Conditional Offer of Employment by the IFD. This offer is contingent on your successful completion of the following requirements:*

1. *Always be fire safe. Know two ways out of every room and have a family meeting place.*
2. *Always use your best crayons when coloring a fire truck picture!*
3. *Always keep your bedroom clean with your fire boots ready for action!*
4. *Make sure the fire hydrant near your house is clear of leaves and snow.*
5. *Get plenty of rest at night so you are always ready for action.*

*The start date of the next full Recruit Class is dependent upon the various remaining testing components, in conjunction with approval by the Public Employees Retirement Fund (PERF) of the state of Indiana. In the meantime, you are to report at 10:30 am for pre-recruit class training on Thursday, January 8, 2015 at IFD Station 13 located at 429 W Ohio St. Indianapolis, IN. Please ask for Captain Tim Robinson when you arrive.*

> *Sincerely,*
> *Ernest Malone, Chief of Fire,*
> *Indianapolis Fire Department*

Laura filmed Jordan opening the letter.

"I got hired!" he shouted, "Thank you, Chief Malone!"[3]

Jordan accepted both job offers and did work days with both

firehouses. He traded in his plastic toy fire helmet for a real one with a big "13" on the front, and a real fireman's jacket with "McLINN" on the back. He even got his own locker stall in the firehouse next to those of all the other firemen where he could hang his gear.

His story got tons of media attention. Local TV news crews came to cover his interviews and first day on the job. And as word spread, more and more firehouses began reaching out to Jordan.

"Firefighters all over the country have just embraced our family and every day it's like there's something new," Laura says. Helmets, patches, T-shirts, and toy trucks started arriving from firehouses coast to coast—Texas, Illinois, Minnesota, Washington State, Alabama, Nevada, and New Jersey, among others—along with invitations to visit.

And in Indianapolis, Laura says, "The whole fire department has basically just embraced our family. We go and eat lunch all the time and Jordan does little trainings and it's just awesome. Like we're just a part of the firefighter family now, and not just one station. It's awesome for Jordan. It's awesome for our whole family."

If it ended there, it would be a nice, heartwarming story—firefighters embrace dying boy and make his dream come true.

But the story didn't end there.

"This, to me, is where the story gets *really* good," Laura says.

One day, Tom Hanify, the president of the Professional Firefighters Union of Indiana, called Laura and said, "Hey, I would like to take you and Jordan on a tour at the statehouse and Jordan can help me do some lobbying for the firefighters."

It seemed like a great opportunity to learn a little about how government works. So Jordan and Laura spent a day at the state capitol with Hanify and Mike Whited of the firefighters union.

"They taught us how to lobby," she says. "They showed us the statehouse. We had lunch with our senator. We met lots of senators and representatives and Jordan walked around in his fire gear. He was actually helping Tom lobby for protecting the pension for the firefighters, something for a training academy, and then also to get a Dalmatian in every firehouse. So that was kind of like just a little fun thing. And the whole day was really just meant to be for fun."

A couple of weeks later, however, one of Laura's neighbors called and said, "Hey, did you see the front page of the *Indianapolis Star*? Have you ever heard of Right to Try?"

There was a big story about how the Indiana legislature was considering a bill to make investigational medicines not yet approved by the FDA available to patients in Indiana with terminal illnesses.

Laura started making calls and found out that the Indiana House Health Committee was holding a hearing that very day. So she and Jordan decided to put their new lobbying skills to work.

"Within a matter of hours, I put together these lobbying sheets, just like Tom Hanify taught us, with Jordan's story on it," she says. "And within hours Jordan and I were standing before the House Health Committee and we were actually testifying about Right to Try and how it might benefit him. Literally within hours I get all this stuff together and we go to the statehouse and they let us testify."

All the news stations that had covered Jordan's interview with the fire department learned what he was doing and started covering Jordan's lobbying campaign.

"We passed out our little papers to everyone that we saw in the statehouse and all the media was there and there are several news stations here that have been following Jordan since the whole Christmas thing and so they did coverage of it. And so the health committee unanimously decided to move it forward."

A week later, Jordan was up in the balcony of the House chamber and got to witness the vote when the House unanimously approved Right to Try.

"Everybody in the room voted yes and it was very emotional," Laura says.

Jordan's work was not over. Now the bill went to the Senate. "We go and we get our sheets together and we start contacting senators and then we actually went and testified before the Senate Health Committee," Laura says.

On March 4, 2015, Jordan walked into the Senate hearing room.

"From the instant Jordan McLinn walked into the Statehouse committee room Wednesday, the 5-year-old made it his own," the news channel Fox 59 reported that day.[4] Dressed in his fire gear, he walked behind the dais and introduced himself to the senators, shaking hands with each one, before joining his mom at the witness table.

My Goldwater colleague Kurt Altman was there to testify as well. Kurt recalls, "In the middle of my testimony, Jordan walks right up to me at the table and starts to tap on the microphone while I'm answering the senators' questions. I kind of chuckled and put my arm around him, and he sat on my lap for the rest of my testimony."

When Jordan's turn to speak came, his mom asked him: "Do you want to say something?"

The bright-eyed boy leaned into the microphone with a big smile, and offered three simple words:

"Please say yes."

They did.

The vote in committee was unanimous and the vote in the full Senate was as well.

Indiana governor Mike Pence invited Jordan to be there when he signed the bill into law. Jordan stood right next to the governor, dressed up in his fire gear, and handed him the pens as he added his signature to the bill.

"I've signed this today with a prayer that the right to try will be a pathway toward healing for Hoosiers for generations to come," Pence declared.[5]

"All the firefighters from the Ladder 13, which is his fire station downtown, they actually surprised us and they all showed up in their dress uniforms," Laura says. "So we were all in there together. Tom Hanify was there from the firefighters union, all the firefighters, and Jordan and our family."

Laura knows Right to Try won't help Jordan in the immediate term. "Right to Try doesn't work unless a drug has made it through the first phase of the FDA. Technically his drug hasn't made it through that first phase, so Right to Try doesn't really apply to Jordan yet," she says. "But we're trying to be proactive and we're trying to raise money to pay for the drug" when it becomes available.

Laura has gotten to know Jenn McNary. "Jenn's kids, they are leading the way, which is awesome for all these boys," she says.

"I knew from the first day that we started this that Jordan might not benefit from Right to Try, but, my God, there're so many people that can, and how incredible is it for him to be a part of maybe saving other people's lives."

That's why Jordan wanted to be a firefighter—to help others.

After Jordan was first diagnosed, Laura had prayed fervently for a miracle. Now she is convinced her prayers are being answered.

"I believe God gives us miracles in many different ways," she says. "Sometimes it can be an instant healing. Sometimes he gives scientists knowledge to create treatments. And sometimes miracles aren't physical in nature at all. I see Jordan's destiny coming into play every day in a new way as we go through this process. He is helping people and giving people hope at just five years old.

"Obviously we hope and pray that something, anything comes through for Jordan," Laura says.

But, she adds, "My dream is for my son to change the world. And that's what Right to Try I think is going to do for Jordan."[6]

"He's going to be able to say, 'I saved a life.'"[7]

Because *that* is what firemen do.

## COLORADO

In Colorado—the first state to pass Right to Try—it was the story of a forty-one-year-old dad with cancer that inspired the Right to Try movement.

In March 2010 Nick Auden went to the doctor and had a cancerous mole removed. He thought the worst was over. But in September 2011 he came home and told his wife, Amy, that he had found a lump under his arm. After going back to the doctor for tests, he learned the devastating news: he had a stage four melanoma that had spread throughout his whole body. He was told he would probably die in less than a year.

At the time, Amy was pregnant with their third child.

Nick beat those odds, and two years later he was still alive, still fighting his cancer. But the tide of the struggle was turning against him. His tumors were growing, the radiation and cancer drugs he was taking had stopped working, and time was running out.

Then one day, his oncologist told him about an emerging treatment called anti-PD-1 immunotherapy. The reason the body's immune system does not attack certain cancers is that the cancer cells have a cloaking mechanism called PD-1, which helps them hide. Scientists had developed anti-PD-1 drugs that stripped away the cloaking mechanism, exposing the cancer to the immune system, which then attacks it.

The anti-PD-1 drugs were being developed by Bristol-Myers Squibb and Merck. Nick immediately tried to get into a clinical trial. Unfortunately, his tumors had spread to his brain. He was told that to qualify for a trial, he had to have no brain tumors or at least ones that were no longer growing. So Nick and his oncologist worked to stop the growth of his brain tumors so he could qualify for the trial.

By July 2013 they had succeeded. Scans showed his brain tumors had stopped growing. Nick was admitted into the Merck clinical trial.

But then disaster struck. Within a few hours of learning that he was admitted, Nick was rushed to the emergency room with a bowel obstruction—a common occurrence for patients with certain advanced cancers. Tests showed he had a perforated intestine. Doctors stabilized him, but the new medical complication disqualified him from the trial again. He would not get the drug he needed to save his life after all.

In the weeks that followed, Amy could not sleep. Lying awake at 3:00 a.m. one night, she decided she was not going to sit back and watch her husband die. They were going to do something. They were going to fight. They were going to get the companies to provide the PD-1 drug under compassionate use.

They petitioned both companies and both turned them down. So Amy launched a website called SaveLockysDad.com. It included a moving video featuring Nick's seven-year-old son, Lachlan "Locky" Auden.

"I love my dad," Locky says, with an adorable gap-toothed grin. "My dad is so strong that he can get better. I want my dad to get the PD-1 drug because then I can do all the things I like to do with him all the time."

Amy looks at the camera and says, "When we were told two weeks ago that this is the end of the road, I can't accept that. Waiting for FDA approval is not going to work either. We can't wait. We need this drug now. And we want you to help us. We want Merck and Bristol-Myers Squibb to help us."[8]

She asked viewers to sign her Change.org petition.

Over 524,000 people did.

But the drug companies did not budge. They assured Nick and Amy they were working as fast as possible to get the drug approved. But time was running short. In October Auden told ABC News, "Not everyone has as short a window as I. Why can't they supply me now rather than me missing by a couple of months? Imagine Amy explaining that to the kids."[9]

He died a month later, on November 22, 2013.

After his death the family issued a statement:

With saddened hearts, we must convey to Nick's hundreds and thousands of supporters that Nick Auden passed away Friday morning with Amy by his side. . . .

This mission is not over. Nick and Amy's fight and your support of them—and in the end, Nick's death—beams a spotlight on a glaring need for change in compassionate access practices for life-saving drugs in late-stage investigational trials.

More on this when the time is right.[10]

The time was right the following year, when the Colorado legislature became the first in the country to consider Right to Try legislation. We had specifically chosen Colorado to be first because it was a state with a Democratic governor and a Democratic legislature. We wanted to make clear from the outset that notwithstanding Goldwater's reputation as a conservative organization, this was a nonpartisan effort.

The bill was cosponsored by Democratic representative Joann Ginal and Republican representative Janak Joshi, two legislators who are generally on opposite sides of most issues. Representative Joshi is an Indian-born physician, who came to America with nothing more than a suitcase and a hundred dollars, and built a successful medical practice in Colorado Springs. Representative Ginal is bioscientist who had worked in the biological and medical fields for more than twenty years, sometimes as a medical liaison for pharmaceutical companies. So both legislators had a professional knowledge of the issues involved, and their opinions carried weight with their colleagues. Their partnership also sent a signal that this effort transcended the usual party lines. (At one point, Representative Ginal told Kurt Altman, "I never thought I'd be partnering up with the Goldwater Institute!")

When the bill came up for a hearing, several groups came out in opposition, including local hospice organizations, whose representatives testified that the bill would hurt patient care (they argued that if you're trying to actively save your life, you wouldn't be eligible for hospice care that you might need). Kaiser Permanente also sent representatives to testify that the law was unnecessary because the FDA already ran an expanded access program, which worked just fine.

So, we encouraged the patients to speak for themselves. One such patient was Lorraine McCartin, who traveled to Colorado all the way from Boston. Lorraine had been diagnosed with stage four breast cancer and had run out of FDA-approved treatment options, when her doctor found an expanded access program for an experimental drug called T-DM1 at Boston's Dana-Farber Cancer Institute. But just before her treatments were about to begin, the program at Dana-Farber shut down. The only way she could get access to the drug was through a clinical trial in Fairfax, Virginia, 465 miles away. She was usually too sick to fly, so her family drove her, every three weeks, back and forth, between Boston and Virginia so she could get the drug— which ended up saving her life. But she had to make the grueling trip over sixteen times, logging about fifteen thousand miles, before the FDA finally allowed her to get the drug in Boston.

Lorraine was still undergoing treatment when Colorado held its hearings, but she insisted on flying out to testify. The hearing was supposed to start at 2:00 p.m., but another controversial bill was on the agenda before it, and the hearing on that bill dragged on late into the night. Kurt Altman, who was there to testify, was worried about Lorraine and tried to convince her to go back to the hotel. She told him, "There is no way that I'm going back. I'm here for this reason, I'm going to testify." And around midnight, she did, explaining to the committee how the current FDA system was failing patients like her. Her strength was inspiring and left legislators in tears.

Nick Auden's widow, Amy, also lobbied for passage. She told the *Denver Post* she believed Merck and Bristol-Myers Squibb did not give Nick the drugs he needed to save his life because they were concerned that if he died while on the drug outside the clinical trial, they would have had to report it to the FDA.

"We needed hope but didn't receive it through our battle. I want others to have opportunities to gain access to medication that can potentially be helpful," she said. Right to Try, she said, "gives patients more of a chance to get the medicines they need, to possibly cure an illness. For the patients, for their families, it offers some hope."[11]

Inspired by stories like Amy and Nick Auden's, and the testimony of survivors like Lorraine, legislators passed the bill unanimously.

Governor John Hickenlooper became the first governor in the nation to sign Right to Try into law. "Patients should be able to try a treatment even though it hasn't been approved if it's an attempt to save their life," Hickenlooper said.

When the nation's first Right to Try law was finally enacted, the *Coloradan* reported that "Nick Auden didn't live to see the legislation, but the case of the Denver melanoma patient who died while seeking access to an experimental drug helped inspire a first-of-its-kind law in Colorado."[12]

The new Colorado law was nothing short of a political miracle: a bill crafted by an organization named after Senator Barry Goldwater passed without a single dissenting vote by a Democratic-controlled legislature, and was signed by a Democratic governor. The signal to Washington should have been crystal clear: at a time when Republicans and Democrats can agree on almost nothing, we are unanimous when it comes to the Right to Try.

And Colorado would be the first of many states where that unanimity would become apparent.

## MISSOURI

As a medical doctor and a representative in the Missouri state legislature, Jim Neely understood firsthand just how important it is to provide patients with quicker access to potentially life-saving treatments. In 2013 his stepdaughter, Kristina, was pregnant with her fifth child when she began experiencing excruciating pains. An ultrasound revealed that she had a tumor, which was soon diagnosed as stage four colon cancer. The cancer had spread to her liver.

Her pregnancy made her ineligible for enrollment in any clinical trials, and liver failure from her rapidly progressing disease left her with even fewer treatment options.

Kristina's plight inspired her stepfather, Jim, to introduce Right to Try legislation that would clear the roadblocks preventing terminal patients from trying to save their own lives.

On February 26, 2014, Jim testified before a Missouri House committee. He choked up as he shared Kristina's story. But, he said, "this is about more than just one patient, it's about guaranteeing the rights of those who are most in need. This legislation offers a beacon of hope for terminal patients who have nowhere else to turn. It's true that we don't know if some of these investigational drugs will work, but we do know they are better than the alternative of simply waiting to die with no hope for a cure."

Neely read aloud from a 2002 *Wall Street Journal* essay by Edie Bacon, a Massachusetts mother who had been diagnosed with a rare and deadly form of cancer called metastatic soft tissue sarcoma.[13] Bacon wrote about her failed effort to get access to an emerging drug called ET-743, owned by Johnson & Johnson. The closest clinical trial was in San Antonio, she wrote, and she was too sick to travel once a week to Texas. So she had asked Johnson & Johnson to give her the drug under compassionate use. The company turned down her request.

"Why?" she wrote. "FDA rules."

According to Bacon,

Any outside use of the drug that cannot be monitored directly by the doctors in charge of the test could "taint" the whole test, if the patient were to experience an unpredicted symptom. The FDA could require more tests, costing Johnson & Johnson millions more in testing costs and delays and hurting its reputation with the FDA.

If you're me, you wonder what the FDA is thinking. I'm dying here; I'm a citizen and a taxpayer. Why must Johnson & Johnson be paralyzed by the prospect of getting in trouble with the government if it gives its drug to dying people? The government wants proof of efficacy before it will allow me to take this drug outside of an approved trial. But the "proof" is years away and I need the drug now. It's safe. It might work. Johnson & Johnson would let me have it if they could do so without the threat of a government hassle. But they're so caught up in the FDA web that the life of an individual patient has no importance whatsoever.

Without ET 743, I'm a dead woman walking. Five kids are going to wonder why they're left without a mother. Won't somebody help me get this drug?

Bacon died three years later. She never got the drug. It is available for use in Europe under the name Yondelis (trabectedin),[14] but it is still not approved here in America. In 2015—*thirteen years* after Bacon made her public appeal—the FDA granted Yondelis priority review.[15] The priority review came too late for the Massachusetts mom.

"I can substitute my daughter for that woman," Neely told the committee, as he put down his copy of the article. "People fighting for their lives shouldn't have to battle red tape. People have a right to determine their future, not the FDA."

Kristina joined her stepfather's campaign for the Right to Try. She was too sick to testify, but she invited PBS *NewsHour* to her home and shared her story. FDA bureaucrats, she said, are "not sitting there counseling me on these medications and what I should do, what I shouldn't do. How to take care of myself to keep myself healthy. And my doctor is. And if my doctor thinks this medication would help me in some way, then that's up to my doctor. That shouldn't be up to somebody that has no involvement in my care."[16]

Kristina's public appeal, Jim Neely's touching testimony, and Edie

Bacon's tragic story inspired a unanimous vote in both chambers of the Missouri legislature in favor of Right to Try. And on July 14, 2014, Democratic governor Jay Nixon signed it into law.[17] "We want to do what we can if people want to get the most up-to-date treatments, to have as few as limitations at the state level to that," Nixon said.

Kristina passed away in April 2015. But thanks to her incredible efforts, and those of her stepfather, other Missourians will now have the Right to Try.

## ILLINOIS

"I am a person who is living with HIV," Illinois state representative Greg Harris says.

"I tested positive early in the epidemic back in the '80s. I'm of a generation where most of the people who are gay men of my age, a lot died back then just because there were no choices available."

He recalls that painful period with deep sadness. "There wasn't even AZT at that time," he says. "Then every once in a while you would hear from a friend or from your doctor, 'Hey, they finally invented a new medicine that might be able to save your life and it's in the testing phase and you might be able to get access to it in a clinical trial.'"

He managed to get into a trial, but he knew many people who didn't.

"Clinical trials are very strictly designed," he says. "I came to learn that there are all kinds of factors that limit your access to it, whether it's your age, any coexisting illnesses, or previous health conditions. There are all these restrictions that you couldn't always get into a clinical trial. But it was the only way you could get access to a drug that could be the only thing that would save your life."

The Oscar-nominated movie *Dallas Buyers Club* told the story of how an AIDS patient diagnosed in the mid-1980s smuggled unapproved drugs into Texas while facing opposition from the FDA. In response to AIDS patients' demands for access to investigational drugs, the FDA began its first formal expanded access—or compassionate use—programs in 1987 to allow limited access to patients outside the clinical-trial setting.

"To this day I cannot watch a movie like that because it just brings up too much emotion for me," Harris says. "I did live it and it's just too distressing for me to have to go back and relive those days, to be really honest—of wondering every day if you were going to survive or if you were going to get some opportunistic infection that would be the end of you."

Harris says that the FDA's compassionate use program, which emerged from the AIDS crisis, is insufficient to meet the needs of Americans fighting terminal illnesses.

"The FDA process is too lengthy and cumbersome for many to complete," he says, "and only a small fraction of those who want access are able to get it. The application alone can take physicians a hundred hours to fill out."

So when Republican state senator Mike Connelly approached him about sponsoring Right to Try legislation in the Illinois House, Harris jumped at the opportunity.

"Having seen so many people die in front of my eyes from . . . just with this one disease, not to mention the people with cancer and MS and other conditions who have struggled knowing that there was something out there that they could not have access to, it was just a perfect opportunity to work on it."

Connelly and Harris made an unlikely pair: a socially conservative Republican and a gay liberal Democrat with HIV. Kurt Altman flew out to Chicago to represent the Goldwater Institute at the press conference at which Connelly and Harris announced they were introducing Right to Try. He says, "Reporters asked me afterward, 'How did you do this? These guys have never been on the same side of any issue, ever.' I told them, 'It's not a Republican or Democratic issue. They're both human beings and this is important to human beings.'" Connelly says his alliance with Harris makes sense, because accessing life-saving treatments is an issue that crosses all ideological lines.

"This is the first bill I've ever encountered that is both pro-life *and* pro-choice," Connelly says. "It gives people the freedom to choose to fight for their life."

Connelly says that he never saw such unanimity as when he approached his colleagues on the Senate floor and asked for their support. "Everybody has had a family friend or neighbor who's gone through some form of terminal illness, and they've seen them fight with everything they have to live."

That includes him. Connelly says his brother-in-law was diagnosed with a glioblastoma around 2006 and was given just a few years to live. "I remember like it was yesterday him sitting up in his hospital bed at Northwestern Memorial Hospital on his computer. And he's already looking at experimental treatments. This is the first day he was diagnosed!

"So he's already thinking, 'Okay, I'm not taking this terminal diagnosis as a final answer. I'm going to do what I have to do.' And that's a natural human reaction. Which is, 'Wait, I'm going to do something myself, I'm going to fight for myself, and I'm going to fight to get better.'"

Kurt testified before both the House and the Senate health committees. In the House, he said, Harris had wrapped up the votes before the hearing even began. "He had talked to everybody. The respect that he commands in that Illinois legislature is pretty cool to see. Literally, the hearing took like four minutes, because he had it all done [in advance]. Everybody votes unanimously—we're done."

In the Senate, the hearing took longer but also went smoothly. Kurt was taking questions from the chairman of the committee. "He's this old guy," Kurt recalls. "Been in the legislature forever and he looks at me and goes, 'Mr. Altman, I have one more question. "Goldwater," is that Barry Goldwater?' I said, 'Mr. Chairman, it is, the institute is named after Senator Barry Goldwater.' He goes, 'Do you have one of them bumper stickers that says "AuH2O," you know, for "Goldwater"?' I said, 'Mr. Chairman, in fact I do have one of those bumper stickers.' He goes, 'You know what my bumper sticker said?' I said, 'No, Mr. Chairman, I do not.' He goes, 'Mine said, "LBJ4USA." I said, 'Well, Mr. Chairman, it certainly appears there were a lot more of those bumper stickers then there were of the ones I have.' He's says, 'Yes indeed there were!' "

The Senate committee passed Right to Try unanimously as well. And thanks to Connelly and Harris's leadership, Right to Try was then approved in the Illinois House by a vote of 114 to 1 and in the Illinois Senate by a vote of 55 to 0.[18]

Asked about his hopes for the new law, Harris says, "I hope this shows that in Illinois, Republicans and Democrats, social liberals and social conservatives, can reach across the aisle to solve problems for suffering families. These families are desperate to cut through red-tape to access possible cures for their loved ones when all other treatments have failed.

"Right to Try is a huge leap forward to help connect our state's most terminal patients with some of the nation's best medical resources, including here in Chicago, and give them the gift of life."[19]

## TEXAS

In 2007 Andrea Sloan was diagnosed with ovarian cancer. A beloved Austin lobbyist who quit her job as a corporate lawyer to run a non-profit that provides free legal services to victims of domestic violence, she underwent two rounds of chemotherapy, five surgeries, and a stem-cell transplant. Nothing worked. The cancer kept coming back.

By 2013 Sloan's oncologist at MD Anderson Cancer Center, Dr. Charles Levenback, told her that her only hope of survival was an experimental drug called BMN-673. The drug, made by the California drug manufacturer BioMarin, inhibits DNA repair in cancer cells and is particularly effective in patients who had a genetic mutation called BRCA—which made it perfect for Sloan.

The drug was not yet approved by the FDA and Sloan did not qualify for a clinical trial. So she and Dr. Levenback tried to get it for her on a compassionate use basis. But BioMarin refused to even look at her medical records or engage her in a dialogue.

It just said "no."

Sloan launched a campaign to convince the company to change its mind, and her many friends in the world of Texas politics rallied around her. They formed what they called "Andi's Army"[20]—a grassroots movement to win access to the drug she needed to save her life. They started a Change.org petition that got 234,837 supporters.[21] Eighty-two Texas state lawmakers petitioned the company on her behalf. Sloan even made a video with a direct plea to BioMarin's CEO, Jean-Jacques Bienaimé.[22]

But the company was unmoved.

Finally, when it became clear BioMarin would not budge, Sloan and her supporters approached another drug company that was developing a similar drug. The company agreed to give Sloan the drug, but asked to do so anonymously.

"It would have been better a few months ago," Dr. Levenback told the *Huffington Post*, expressing frustration with BioMarin's refusal to share its version of the drug.[23] "The point is it's cancer. If you don't do anything, it gets worse."

Once the company agreed to provide the drug, Sloan faced another delay when she had to seek FDA approval to take it. Dr. Levenback had to spend over one hundred hours on Andrea's application. Then, says Andrea's best friend, Michelle Wittenberg, a lobbyist, it took nearly a month to get FDA approval for an expanded access petition, during which time her health deteriorated. "We waited twenty-four days for the FDA to give their approval," she says. "It took them twenty-four days to process an application. That's really problematic because I saw her every day and she did deteriorate on a daily basis during that twenty-four-day period.

"She would say, 'Michelle, what's going on? What's the delay? The drug company's agreed to give it, why is it taking so long? The FDA said they didn't have a problem, why is it taking so long? What do we do?'"

When the FDA finally cleared the way for Sloan to get the drug, a miracle happened. The drug actually worked—scans showed it was beating back the cancer. "She had scans that were done in her body in July that had black spots, i.e., cancer that showed up prevalently," Wittenberg says. "And then she had scans on December 16 after taking the drug for two and a half months. We got the results of those scans on December 18 and her parents were there, I was there, Andrea was there, her medical team was there—Dr. Levenback in the lead and another gentleman who's one of the heads of the Moonshot program for ovarian cancer at MD Anderson. And I've never in my life seen a more giddy group of physicians. It was a turnaround. They put the scans up against each other and, oh, it was unbelievable. It's like, where are the black spots? They're gone. We got the scan, it was *glorious*, *amazing*, *amazing* improvement. She was weak, but everything was on the upward trajectory and just was amazing."

Then, a few days after getting the scans, Sloan suffered a setback when she came down with pneumonia. "And thirteen days later, she was dead," Wittenberg says. "Her system wasn't strong enough to fight it off." She died on New Year's Day 2014—just two weeks after learning that the drug was beating back the cancer.

The terrible injustice was that, based on her response to the drug, if she had gotten access sooner, it might well have saved her life. "It wasn't just the disease, it was the delay that killed her," Wittenberg says. "The delay in getting that drug, that was working, killed her. Three months' waiting is too long. Two months' waiting was too long. The extra month tacked on because of the FDA process, too long. And that should be unconscionable to anybody.

"I will say this about the FDA, they wanted to help Andrea," Wittenberg says. But she cannot understand the reason for the twenty-four-day delay. "You look at their website and it says they can process an emergency application in a day. Well, this was an emergency. How come it took almost a month? When somebody's life is on the line, your bureaucratic process helped contribute to the cost of a life. That would weigh on me."

Andi had died, but Andi's Army didn't disband. Quite the opposite: her friends kept the movement alive, and deployed it to fight a new fight—to pass the Right to Try law in Texas.

Wittenberg was doing some research on compassionate use reform when she came across the Goldwater Institute's website and read about Right to Try. "I looked online and sent a blind email to someone at the Goldwater Institute," she says. She connected with Victor Riches and Kurt Altman, who walked her through the law and how it was handled in other states. "I was kind of a hard sell," she says. This was her best friend's legacy and she wanted to do right by Andrea. But once she became convinced that Right to Try was the right thing to do, she rallied Andi's Army behind it and swung into action.

"There were two state legislators who are about my age and Andrea's age, forty-four years old—their names are Ken King and Kyle Kacal," Wittenberg says. "Their mothers had both died of ovarian cancer within the past year. And we were all good friends and they knew Andrea and watched what she went through too." Wittenberg told them about Right to Try, and they became the principal sponsors of what became known as the "Andrea Sloan Right to Try Act."

"We hit our 150 members in the Texas house, and over 100 signed on as coauthors, which is not common," Wittenberg says. "The senate bill had over twenty authors, and there are only thirty-one Texas senators."

Victor Riches remembers Wittenberg as a legislative force of nature. "I went out there to meet with the legislators and she literally set up meetings with thirty legislators over about a forty-eight-hour period. She was very passionate about it."

"She asked us to Texas probably four or five times," Kurt Altman recalls. "Texas's statehouse is just huge and it's very confusing with all these different levels. I was lost all the time. And Michelle would always be fifteen yards in front of me, and I would lose her in the crowd she'd be so fast. She was on a mission, and she would be marching and literally I would be sweating every day because I'd have to chase her through the statehouse."

In meetings, Kurt recalls, "she would start to talk about Andrea Sloan somehow and at least once or twice a day she would start to tear up and it would just kill me and she'd look at me and go, 'Stop, stop, I told you I wasn't going to do this.' We'd always be in front of a senator or somebody who knew her, and he would say, 'Now, Michelle, it's all right.' She'd wipe her tear away and say, 'We're good, you just make sure that we get this through, this is important.' She was very inspirational. She's such a go-getter, and there was no way if I was ever tired that I'd be able to stop when I was with her."

The Texas legislature meets only every other year, for a very short session, so the window of opportunity to move the legislation was short. Wittenberg was not going to wait two years to try again—she was determined to pass the law immediately.

Wittenberg testified before the Texas Senate Committee on Health and Human Services, as did Sloan's physician, Dr. Levenback, and Sloan's parents. Andrea's mother, Karen Sloan, spoke movingly of her daughter's fight to save her life and of the FDA's unconscionable delays. "Twenty-four days is a lifetime for people who are terminally ill," she told the committee.

Their efforts paid off. On May 22, 2015, the Texas state senate unanimously passed the Andrea Sloan Right to Try Act, and the Texas assembly soon approved it unanimously as well.

At the bill-signing ceremony, Sloan's oncologist, Dr. Levenback, took Wittenberg aside and asked if there was any way he could get a formal copy of the new law. "He said, 'I'd like to get a copy of the bill and a picture of Andrea and have it framed, and I want to put it out in the waiting room.' He said, 'People should know what she did. I want our patients to know.'"

She got him a copy, and the Right to Try law now occupies a place of honor on the wall outside his office at MD Anderson Cancer Center.

"The spread of these laws shows the level of public dissatisfaction with this part of the medical economy," Dr. Levenback told the *Houston Chronicle*. "It just seems fundamentally not right to put so much time and money into drug development, to brag about this great health care system that produces such great medical innovations, and then for it to prove so difficult for deserving patients to get new drugs.

"We deserve better," he said.[24]

Thanks to Andrea Sloan and the soldiers in Andi's Army, deserving patients in Texas will now have the chance to get better.

They now have the Right to Try.

## VIRGINIA

When a Virginia boy named Josh Hardy was just nine months old, he was diagnosed with kidney cancer. The tumor on his left kidney was the size of a softball, and the one on the right was the size of a walnut.

He underwent ten rounds of chemotherapy, six days of radiation, and surgery to remove the tumors.[25] He beat the cancer, but it came back three times as he grew—returning in his thymus, lung, and bone marrow. Each time he beat it back, but the treatments took a toll on his system.

In January 2014 doctors told his parents, Todd and Aimee Hardy, that Josh had developed a bone-marrow disorder that often follows intensive cancer treatments. He needed a bone-marrow transplant.

So they took him to St. Jude Children's Research Hospital in Memphis for the surgery.

After undergoing the transplant, Josh experienced heart failure; he had to be put on a ventilator and was in a coma for sixteen days. His doctors had to give Josh special drugs to suppress his immune system so that his body would not reject the new bone marrow. While his immune system was compromised, Josh developed a life-threatening adenovirus infection that spread throughout his body. Doctors tried an FDA-approved antiviral drug, cidofovir, but it caused complications with his kidneys and had to be stopped.

Josh was dying.

Josh's doctors at St. Jude said the only hope for Josh was an antiviral drug called brincidofovir. The drug was being developed by a North Carolina company called Chimerix. They believed it would work for Josh because they had participated in some of the clinical trials, and had seen brincidofovir clear up adenovirus in children in two weeks.

"Our doctor said they had done an adenovirus study at St. Jude's, and in every child that had been a part of that study they had suppressed the adenovirus," Aimee Hardy says. "So he's like, 'I really want this medicine for him.'"

But there was a problem: Josh did not qualify for a clinical trial, because the drug was being tested only in adults at that point. They would have to ask the company to provide the drug on a compassionate use basis.

On February 12 Josh's doctors at St. Jude called Chimerix and asked for permission to use the drug. The company said no. It had once had a compassionate use program but had discontinued it, deciding to focus instead on accelerating FDA approval.

Chimerix would not provide the drug.

Josh's parents were stunned.

After consulting with his doctors, they decided to try again. His doctors composed an email explaining Josh's circumstance, why they believed the drug would save him, and the case for giving Josh access to the drug. An executive wrote back by email saying that Chimerix was not "in a position to provide drug for this and other subjects in similar circumstances due to a limited inventory and our limited resources."

"The company kept saying no, no, no," Aimee says.

They had hit a dead end.

With Josh barely hanging on to life, his parents had little to lose. So they decided to make their fight public. They launched a Facebook and Twitter campaign with the hashtag #savejosh and asked people to tweet, email, and call the company. The campaign went viral. Thousands of strangers rallied around Josh and the fight to save his life.

"We were just brainstorming, like, who do we know that might have some influence with the company or something? And then we thought, we don't know anybody," Aimee says. "We put it out on Facebook and it turns out we know a lot of people. It was just an amazing thing to find out how many people really support us."

When one of Josh's cousins, Regina Breedlove, launched a Change .org petition, it got nearly twenty thousand signatures in a matter of days. The Washington Redskins quarterback Robert Griffin III urged his 1.3 million Twitter followers to join the crusade to #savejosh.[26] People flooded the company with calls and emails demanding that it give the drug to Josh. They simply could not believe that the company would let a boy die of an illness that was entirely curable.

Soon, national news organizations picked up Josh's story. On March 11, 2014, CNN ran a spot titled "Company Denies Drug to Dying Child."[27] The network reported:

In an intensive care unit in Memphis, a virus ravages the body of a 7-year-old who's in heart and kidney failure. He vomits blood several times an hour as his family gathers in vigil.

In a cabinet in Durham, North Carolina, there's a drug that could likely help Josh Hardy, but the drug company won't give it to him. They're adamant that spending the time to help Josh and others like him will slow down their efforts to get this drug on the market. . . .

When asked how he will feel if Josh dies—and he's in critical condition, so sadly that could happen soon—the president of the company that makes the drug doesn't hesitate to answer.

"Horrible," said Kenneth Moch [the company's CEO]. He would feel horrible and heartbroken.

But still, he said there's no way he's going to change his mind. There's no way he's going to give Josh this drug.

The Hardys kept up the pressure. Fox News and other networks aired the company's phone number and email address on screen, prompting thousands of calls and messages.

As pressure mounted, the company protested that it had only fifty employees and could not afford to provide the drug to everyone who wanted it on a compassionate basis. But that excuse evaporated when it emerged that Chimerix had received $72 million in federal funds.[28]

Then, a private charity, the Max Cure Foundation, stepped forward and offered to cover the costs of Josh's treatment. "I spoke to Mr. Moch yesterday by phone," Richard Plotkin, the vice chair of Max Cure, told Peter Johnson Jr., Fox News' chief medical correspondent. "I told him that we had the $50,000 that I thought he was claiming he needed to supply the drug. He then told me it isn't about money. He told me it's all about ethics."[29] Plotkin said he asked Moch what he would do if it were his child or grandchild. Moch, he said, hung up on him.

When Fox News emailed a member of Chimerix's board of directors, Tim Wollaeger, and asked whether the board would give the drug to Josh, he answered, "Don't you people realize there is an FDA? We have done what we can. Say a prayer for Josh."[30]

In fact, thousands of Americans *were* praying for Josh—and

tweeting, and emailing, and calling, and writing, and demanding that Chimerix do the right thing.

Eventually those prayers were answered. After days of public shaming, Chimerix finally relented. It opened a special twenty-person clinical trial for children and agreed to admit Josh as the first patient.

His mom, Aimee, posted the news on Facebook: "Glory to GOD! They are releasing the drug for Josh!!!!!"

Within days of receiving the drug, Josh began to make a remarkable recovery. The level of adenovirus in his blood dropped from 250,000 copies per millimeter to 367 copies per millimeter. On March 31, the family celebrated Josh's eighth birthday—a milestone that seemed unreachable just a few days earlier.

In April Moch stepped down as CEO of Chimerix.

In July, after six and a half months at St. Jude, Josh finally went home. He was not yet able to go to school or spend a lot of time in public places, because of the danger of contracting another virus. But he got tutoring at home, and he was able to play video games with his siblings and ride his bike on the street in front of their house.

When a local news channel visited the Hardy family after Josh's return, Aimee talked about her dreams for Josh. "I want him to play baseball and slide home after he hits a great hit, and go to school, go on family vacations and dive in the ocean waves. The whole nine yards."[31]

Josh had slightly different dreams. He wanted to go to Chuck E. Cheese and a Washington Wizards game. A year later, he got his wish when the Wizards invited him to sit courtside for their game against his other favorite team, the Memphis Grizzlies—from the hometown of the doctors who saved him at St. Jude Children's Research Hospital.

As Josh got better, Aimee started hearing from other patients who had received the drug as a result of their campaign.

"Afterward I had a little seventeen-year-old girl message me on Facebook and she had had a liver transplant and she had developed the adenovirus," Aimee says. "When we got ours she was able to get it as well. And she said that she thanked her doctor for getting it and he said, 'Don't thank me. Thank Josh Hardy's family, because they're the reason that you have access to it. You would have never gotten it otherwise.' And that was kind of neat to know that that helped another family. And apparently it's helped about seventy other families."

Indeed, instead of limiting the new trial to twenty patients, Chimerix made it open-ended. And that decision not only helped save dozens of other lives but led Chimerix to seek additional FDA approval for the drug in the pediatric indication Josh presented.

Aimee and Todd wanted to help make sure other kids did not have to face the same struggles to get life-saving treatments that Josh did. That opportunity soon presented itself.

Josh's parents grew up in Virginia's Richmond County with Todd Ransone, whose wife, Margaret, just happened to be a member of the Virginia House of Delegates.

"I actually grew up playing with Margaret's husband," Aimee says. "They were neighbors of family members and they knew us very closely, and so she was impacted emotionally" by Josh's plight.

"I had a son the exact same age," Ransone says. "I vowed to that mom I'm going to do everything that I can to research this and see what we can do." She did some research and saw that Colorado had recently passed a Right to Try bill. So she teamed up with state senator Bryce Reeves—whose son plays lacrosse with Josh's brother—to introduce the Right to Try Act in the Virginia General Assembly.

Josh became the public face of the fight to pass Right to Try in Virginia. Aimee testified before the health committees in the Virginia House and Senate, lobbied legislators, and held press conferences as the bill wound its way through the legislature.

Standing in the briefing room of the capitol, she shared the story of her family's fight to save Josh. "That's what was also really maddening to me—that he could survive cancer four times, and have a simple virus take him down." she said. "Having to leave their bedside while they are in the ICU to fight for a drug is just—it's just it shouldn't happen."[32]

"You need to not have to go on national TV or beg people to call the company for you or do all these things," she said. "Everyone should just have the right to try."[33]

Aimee was joined in her campaign for the Right to Try by Frank Burroughs, a Virginian who had faced a similar situation fourteen years earlier when his college-age daughter Abigail developed head and neck cancer.

"She had run out of FDA-approved options in her battle to save her life and we were trying to get the drug Erbitux for her," he says. Abigail did not qualify for clinical trials. The company had studies for colon cancer under way at the time, but Abigail's cancer was in her head and neck. "She had the right cancer cells in the wrong part of her body so that ruled out any chance at a clinical trial."

The company, ImClone, refused to provide the drug on a compassionate use basis. So, just like the Hardys, Frank Burroughs and his daughter launched a campaign to get it to change its mind. This was in 2001, before the age of social media, so there was no Twitter or Facebook or Change.org petition to rally supporters to their cause. But Frank got stories in the *Washington Post* and the local ABC News affiliate.

Sadly, it wasn't enough.

"We weren't able to get the drug," Frank says. "She died on Saturday, June 9, 2001."

About ten hours after she died, amid his unspeakable grief, Frank Burroughs had an epiphany.

"The thought just flashed into my head," he says. "Why should I quit now? There are other people as precious as Abigail."

Eleven days after Abigail's death, Frank testified before the Virginia House Government Reform Committee.[34] He told the legislators:

My only child, dear, sweet, loving, talented and compassionate
Abigail, died at 2:30 p.m. two Saturdays ago, June 9th. The loss of
my beautiful compassionate child has left a hole in my life. . . .

Abigail was an Echols honor student at the University of
Virginia. Abigail cleaned toilets and changed beds in men's
homeless shelters. Abigail worked in a poor neighborhood in
Syracuse, NY, fixing up houses and running a free day camp for
inner city children. Abigail started a major tutoring program for
middle school children who were having learning problems. . . .
The world has lost a brilliant young woman who would have
done great things.

I am here today because the issue of the wider use of compassionate use of drugs is a very important issue, because it touches
tens of thousands of lives. Compassionate Abigail wants us to keep
this issue alive, although we could not keep Abigail alive. . . .

Abigail is now in the arms of God. . . . With the strength of
Abigail's memory, beautiful memory . . . I will keep this issue
alive so others may have a chance to live, a chance that Abigail,
compassionate Abigail, did not have.

With that, the Abigail Alliance for Better Access to Developmental
Drugs was born.

Burroughs has spent the last fourteen years fighting to save the lives
of children like Abigail, and he has turned the Abigail Alliance into a
force to be reckoned with. He has pushed for the accelerated approval
of a number of cancer drugs. He sued the FDA demanding access to
experimental drugs on constitutional grounds. He worked with members of Congress to introduce the Compassionate Access Act of 2005, a
bill he says "never went anywhere." But he did succeed in lobbying for
reforms in the Food and Drug Administration Safety and Innovation
Act (FDASIA Act) in 2012 to create the new "breakthrough therapy"
designation that allows faster approval of novel drugs treating unmet

needs. He works every day with patients to guide them through the FDA's bureaucracy when they seek compassionate use.

And today he's fighting for Right to Try laws.

"Meeting Frank Burroughs, I mean I was heartbroken to hear his story," Aimee says. "I just can't imagine to have that drug out there and then just a couple of years later it's available."

They teamed up to lobby Virginia legislators. Frank joined Aimee Hardy at the capitol building in Richmond to urge them to pass Right to Try.

"The Virginia 'Right to Try' bill is an important part of paving the way for much needed and very doable change at the FDA that will save lives," he said. "In Virginia and other states that have passed 'Right to Try' laws there is broad public support for this change."[35]

Margaret Ransone, the bill's sponsor, was a force to be reckoned with. Kurt Altman recalls her lobbying tactics: "She literally marched me to fifteen or twenty different offices. She'd walk in and say, 'Can we get ten minutes of your time?' She'd lay it out for whoever it was. She'd introduce me, I'd answer all their questions. And then she'd look them right in the eye and say, 'So I need to know right now, are you with me? Are you with me?' And they were funny. They all were taken aback. Most of these meetings end up with, 'Okay, well, I appreciate the information,' and then you leave. We would not leave an office until she got an answer from whomever we talked to. 'Are you with me? I need to know if you're with me. Did I tell you why I did this? Because my friend is the mother of Josh Hardy. Josh would have died. I just need to know, where are you? 'Cause I need to know what else I have to do. Are you with me?' They'd say, 'Margaret I think this is a great idea. Yeah, Margaret, I'm with ya. I'm with ya.' It must have happened twenty times."

Between Aimee Hardy's and Frank Burroughs's heartrending stories, and Delegate Ransone's relentless lobbying, Virginia legislators got the message.

In January 2015 the Virginia House voted 99 to 0 in favor of Right to Try, and the Senate approved it 39 to 0 the following month.

In March Democratic governor Terry MacAuliffe signed it into law.

When Right to Try passed, Aimee Hardy was elated. "We are super excited that hopefully families won't have to experience what we went through," she told reporters.

She simply does not understand people who oppose the Right to Try.

"When you're on that last train out and there's a little glimmer of hope and you're being told you can't even try it, you should be able to have the right to try," she says. When she hears pharmaceutical executives like Ken Moch say that giving the drug to Josh could make it harder to save future Joshes, "I'm like, well, what's wrong with saving Josh right now?" she says.

Aimee acknowledged that Right to Try did not solve all the problems related to reforming compassionate use but she said, "It's a step in the right direction."[36]

"The whole system needs to be reformed. And this is a great start."[37]

Frank Burroughs agrees.

"What is so huge about the Right to Try legislation in Virginia and the other states where it's passed is that it paves the way for changes at the national level," Burroughs says. "People have said this Right to Try law is not going to do much," he says. "And I always say, well that's just not true—absolutely not true. What's happening is it's elevating this issue further. We've seen a pattern here. [It has passed in] every state [where] it's been introduced. [It's] batting a thousand. What this clearly shows is that the vast majority of the public is behind this. So that's what's huge about this bill. And that message is being heard at the FDA and the message is being heard on Capitol Hill.

"The last time I checked, this is a democracy," he says.

. . . .

IN OTHER STATES, THE story was the same.

In Utah, seven-year-old Bertrand Might, a boy with a rare genetic disease called NGLY1, was the face of the local Right to Try movement. Bertrand joined Governor Bob Herbert as he signed Right to Try into law. "Thanks for helping out, buddy, you got legislation passed," Herbert told him.

In Michigan, Terry Kalley championed Right to Try along with his wife, Arlene, who is in her fourth year battling stage four breast cancer. "Of course there are risks," Terry Kalley told lawmakers, "but by far the greatest risk to my wife and her fellow terminally ill patients is not to have access to these drugs. Without access, her risk of death increases to 100 percent."[38] Lawmakers responded by passing the Right to Try by a margin of 109 to 0 in Michigan's House and 31 to 2 in its Senate, and Governor Rick Snyder signed it into law.[39]

In Minnesota, Republican state Representative Nick Zerwas championed Right to Try. Zerwas was born with a three-chambered heart and survived thanks only to experimental surgery that removed the right side of his heart and replaced it with a cow's pericardium. "That was my right to try," the thirty-four-year-old Republican from Elk River told the floor. "We gave it a shot and we got it right."[40] He introduced Right to Try legislation, which passed the Minnesota House 123 to 0 and was signed into law by Democratic governor Mark Dayton.

In Alabama, a ten-year-old boy named Gabe Griffin with Duchenne muscular dystrophy inspired legislators to pass Right to Try. On June 3, 2015, Governor Robert Bentley signed Alabama's Senate Bill 357, the Gabe's Right to Try Act. "Gabe Griffin is a special child who has worked hard to advocate for this legislation," Governor Bentley said. "As a physician, I believe it is extremely important to give terminally ill patients the option to consider experimental treatments. Gabe's story has touched many lives. I appreciate the Alabama Legislature passing this bill and giving Gabe and other children like him hope for the future."[41]

In North Dakota, it was three brothers—Lane, Tanner, and Ty Kulsrud—who suffer from a rare metabolic disorder called PKAN that is leaving deadly iron deposits in their brains.[42] They were joined in supporting the law by the president of the State Bar Association of North Dakota. During the legislative hearings in Bismarck, my colleague Craig Handzlik was preparing to testify when the president was testifying in favor of Right to Try. "He's saying North Dakotans need this, especially the rural folks who would not have access to clinical trials and would have to travel long distances," Craig recalls. "He seems fairly knowledgeable about Right to Try and he finishes his testimony, thanks the committee, and turns around from the podium, looks at me, and says, in front of the whole galley, 'Goldwater Institute, huh? You guys are suing me, asshole.'"

Craig had to call back to the office to ask: Why are were suing the state bar association? We had just filed a suit against them for misusing mandatory dues for political lobbying purposes (we prevailed). It just goes to show, Craig says, that "Right to Try originated with the Goldwater Institute, but it is so widely supported that even folks we are suing will stand up and testify to support it."

In Mississippi, a woman with ALS named Janet Champion and her husband, Sid, spoke out in favor of Right to Try.[43] And, of course, in Arizona it was Diego Morris, the boy we met in chapter 2 who moved to London to get the medicine to cure his osteosarcoma, who led the charge for Right to Try.

Powered by these and other stories of hope and heartbreak, the Right to Try movement is sweeping the nation. Here are the results so far:

Arkansas: 96–0 in the House and 33–0 in the Senate.

Colorado: 65–0 in the House and 35–0 in the Senate.

Indiana: 92–0 in the House and 50–0 in the Senate.

Louisiana: 96–0 in the House and 37–0 in the Senate.

Michigan: 109–0 in the House and 31–2 in the Senate.

Mississippi: 118–0 in the House and 50–0 in the Senate.

Missouri: 143–0 in the House and 26–0 in the Senate.

Montana: 93–7 in the House and 50–0 in the Senate.

Oklahoma: 96–0 in the House and 44–0 in the Senate.

South Dakota: 61–1 in the House and 32–0 in the Senate.

Utah: 69–3 in the House and 26–0 in the Senate.

Wyoming: 58–1 in the House and 28–1 in the Senate.

North Dakota: 91–0 in the House and 42–5 in the Senate.

Minnesota: 123–0 in the House and 60–4 in the Senate.

Florida: 113–0 in the House and 39–1 in the Senate.

Illinois: 114–1 in the House and 55–0 in the Senate.

Texas: 134–0 in the House and 31–0 in the Senate.

Virginia: 99–0 in the house and 39–0 in the Senate.

Alabama: 97–0 in the House and 29–0 in the Senate.

Nevada: 41–0 in the House and 20–0 in the Senate.

Tennessee: 95–0 in the House and 31–0 in the Senate.

North Carolina:118–0 in the House and 47–0 in the Senate.

Oregon: 60–0 in the House and 29–0 in the Senate.

And that's not counting Arizona, where over one million people voted for Right to Try at the ballot box, a pro vote of more than 75 percent.

Put it all together, and in 24 states there have been 3,045 votes in favor or Right to Try and a grand total of 26 votes against. This means Right to Try has been approved in the states where it has come up by a margin of 99 to 1 percent. That's about as close to unanimity as you will ever achieve in a democracy.

And more states are at bat. Right to Try laws have been introduced in Alaska, California, Connecticut, Delaware, Georgia, Hawaii, Kansas, Kentucky, Maine, Massachusetts, New Hampshire, New Jersey, New York, Pennsylvania, Rhode Island, West Virginia, and Wisconsin. In many of these states, the law has already been approved in committee and is awaiting floor action.

The critics of Right to Try say legislators are uninformed and are being manipulated by heartbreaking stories. My colleague Victor Riches, who spearheaded the first days of Right to Try, sees it differently. "This is the kind of issue that comes around maybe once in a lifetime, when you have an issue that really strikes a chord across the country. And once we got it going, it really started moving like wildfire. And it wasn't a Republican issue, wasn't a Democrat issue, it was literally just a human being issue."

Here is a thought for the critics: when you are losing a debate 99 to 1, maybe it's time for some introspection.

There is a reason Americans are instinctively siding with Jordan McLinn, Nick Auden, Andrea Sloan, Josh Hardy, Abigail Burroughs, and all the other patients who are demanding their Right to Try. Most of us have lost a loved one to a terminal illness or know someone who has. As Americans, we believe in fairness. We believe in opportunity. We believe in compassion. We all want the chance to save our lives if we need it.

The patients, legislators, and voters of these states have a message for the government:

We are the 99 percent.

We demand change, and we will get it.

Because Frank Burroughs is right: this *is* still a democracy.

# 7.

# Compassionate Use

*The Mythical Unicorn*

———

The FDA often cites its compassionate use program as the reason why Right to Try laws are unnecessary. Richard Klein, the director of the FDA's patient liaison program, says, "The agency has a pathway. It seems to work quite well, and I'm not sure what the state Right to Try bills really add to that."[1]

Except that it doesn't work so well. Just ask the hundreds of thousands of Americans who are stymied each year in their efforts to get the drugs they need to save their lives.

The FDA's indifference helps explain why the Right to Try movement has taken off in just a year. The agency has buried its head in the sand. Its expanded access system is badly broken. Not only has the FDA created obstacles for patients and doctors seeking access to new treatments, but the agency has also created a system that discourages drug companies from offering innovative treatments on a compassionate basis.

Right to Try laws are a critical part of the solution. But if we are going to make innovative medicines available to all who need them, we also need to change the FDA—by removing obstacles to compassionate use and creating new incentives for manufacturers to do the right thing and help dying Americans who are fighting for their lives.

Americans like Mikaela Knapp.

. . . .

LATE ONE NIGHT, WHILE his wife, Mikaela, lay dying from kidney cancer in her Northern California hospital bed, Keith Knapp opened his email to find a cryptic message that seemed like something out of a spy novel.

"Keith and Mikaela," the message began, "I created this email account to share some information with you. It isn't secret information, but my employers might not appreciate me disseminating it. My wife thought it best to be an anonymous helper right now."

The nameless writer had seen Keith and Mikaela on *Good Morning America* making a public plea for access to an experimental drug that was her last hope—anti-PD-1 immunotherapy, the same treatment Nick Auden tried and failed to gain access to.

The drug was being developed by three pharmaceutical companies—Merck, Bristol-Myers Squibb, and Genentech—but still had not received final FDA approval.

Mikaela had spent six months being treated by doctors at the University of California–San Francisco Medical Center and had tried every approved drug or treatment. She underwent gamma knife radiation treatment for the cancer that had spread to her brain, and both whole brain and spinal radiation treatment. Nothing worked. The cancer had spread to her lungs, making it difficult for her to breathe.

Mikaela tried to get into clinical trials for all of the three anti-PD-1 drugs, but she did not qualify. For one thing, she had the wrong kind of cancer—kidney cancer, not melanoma, which was the focus of the trials. Second, her cancer had spread to her brain, and this disqualified her as a study subject. Like most cancer patients in America, she did not qualify for a clinical trial.

"This drug that we wanted, for some reason they don't want people with brain mass," Keith says. "They want a very standardized sample, they want people who have very localized spreads at worst. So when you start getting people with brain mass and different kind of peculiar circumstances, it can skew their results—which is weird to me because then once the drug is approved it gets used on those people all the same, so it's kind of a strange way to do things."

Eventually Mikaela and Keith went to an oncologist at Stanford University Medical Center for a second opinion. She told them that since Mikaela had run out of approved treatment options and could not get into a clinical trial, she could seek compassionate use of the anti-PD-1 drug under the FDA's expanded access program.

To qualify, Keith says, "you need a doctor willing to administer [the drug] and then the drug company willing to provide the drug."

They had the doctor. Now they needed a drug company.

"The Stanford doctor said she'd be willing to supervise the treatment," Keith says. "So we asked Merck and Bristol-Myers Squibb and Genentech if they would provide their version of the drug."

Bristol-Myers Squibb said its drug was still too early in the development process. Genentech said it did not have enough of the drug to supply it outside clinical trials. Merck was the closest to bringing its version of the drug to market, so Keith and Mikaela focused their efforts on Merck.

When they told Mikaela's original doctor at UC–San Francisco they were seeking compassionate use, Keith says, "he seemed kind of frustrated that we found out about it. What was really frustrating was that they had the drug right there in the hospital where she was being treated where he worked. His direct colleagues were running clinical trials of the drug we wanted."

The drug she needed was right there, but Mikaela could not get access to it.

One night, Mikaela was rushed to the emergency room. Keith looked at his high school sweetheart lying there in the ICU, tubes and wires attached to her body. They had been married just two years and already he was losing her. She was running out of time.

He asked Mikaela what she wanted to do. He would have understood if she decided to stop and just make the most of the time they had left.

But Mikaela said she wanted to fight.

Keith had read about the case of Josh Hardy, the young Virginia boy who survived cancer but needed an experimental drug to fight a life-threatening infection. After being repeatedly turned down, Josh's parents launched a social media campaign to convince the manufacturer to give him the drug. It worked. Josh got the drug and got better.

Inspired by Josh's success, Keith contacted some of Mikaela's friends and former colleagues from her days working in public relations and asked them for help.

"They were able to get us up on some Bay Area blogs and it kind of just took off from there," he says.

Mikaela's friends started a Facebook page with the title "We Got This" and a Twitter account with a hashtag #WeGotThis. "Help Mikaela live beyond 25," they pleaded. They also started an online petition at Change.org with a message from Keith: "We fully understand the risks with experimental medicine, but we have nothing to lose and much to gain."[2] To his astonishment, the petition quickly gathered nearly half a million supporters.

A GiveForward.com fund-raising page raised $19,000 to help Mikaela get the genetic testing she needed to prove the drug could help her. They recorded a YouTube video of Mikaela from her hospital bed making an impassioned plea for access.

The campaign was heartbreaking for Keith. Every time he left Mikaela's bedside for a TV interview or a meeting, he knew it could be the last time he saw her alive. But she wanted to fight, so fight he did.

Within a few short weeks, their story was all over the news. Keith was approached by Frank Burroughs of the Abigail Alliance, who gave him advice on his efforts to convince one of the drug companies to give Mikaela the drug and told him that the Abigail Alliance could help them guide it through the FDA approval process if the drug company agreed.

Soon, Keith and Mikaela were on *Good Morning America*.

"Mikaela's always been my rock. You know, she's in a lot of pain. She's facing death at age 25. She's just such a fighter," Keith told correspondent Jim Avila.

"We just need someone to say that they are going to provide us the drug."[3]

Little did he know his public appeal had touched the heart of someone on the inside.

Shortly after his *GMA* appearance, Keith got the anonymous email. "I am a proponent of compassionate use of investigational drugs and your story drew my extreme interest for a specific reason—I am a Merck employee who works on the anti-PD-1 antibody every day," the source wrote him from a secret email account. "I have seen the amazing clinical results from our melanoma trials, and I am well aware of the multiple cancer types that could be treated with our drug."

Merck could help them if it chose to, the anonymous informant told Keith. "Merck should have plenty of their drug to spare for one person—as an employee, I've followed the dramatic scaling up of production for this antibody over the last year plus."

But he explained the reason why they were facing such resistance. "As you have experienced already, this is going to be a difficult drug to get companies to allow compassionate use. The anti-PD-1 drugs hold the promise of billions of dollars a year in revenue. Merck, Bristol-Myers, and Genentech are all going to be very hesitant to allow the drug to be used outside of the controlled and predictable clinical trials. If this drug were to cause complications while being used with Mikaela, the companies would be worried about that association with their drug."

If Mikaela died while she was on the drug, he explained, the company was afraid the FDA could halt the trial and force it to prove that the disease, and not the drug, was responsible for her death. That could lead to delays in drug approval that could cost it a fortune.

There was no incentive for the company to help Mikaela—and every incentive for it not to help her.

The source gave Keith advice on how to build pressure on the company, revealing the little-known location of the Merck lab where researchers were working on the drug Mikaela needed.

"The address is 901 S. California Avenue, Palo Alto, CA 94304," he wrote. "There is a big Merck sign right out front—a decent backdrop for a rally."

Keith said he needed help figuring out whom to contact at Merck to make his plea. "It was pretty much a black box for us," he said. So the source gave Keith the direct numbers of top Merck executives.

"I want to wish you two the best from the bottom of my heart," he wrote. "I wish we could have been faster in our work so you wouldn't be having to go through this additional struggle. Let me know if you need any additional help. Don't give up and enjoy every moment together."

Keith and his anonymous source began exchanging emails. And they eventually met up at a Starbucks near Merck's Palo Alto lab to strategize.

"He was just kind of telling me about how critical this drug was to Merck, how this is the best hope they've had since the '80s, and really their entire business is dependent on this drug working out," Keith says.

"They had been saying that they couldn't give her the drug because they didn't know the dosing schedule and they didn't know the risks with her situation," Keith says.

His source told him that this wasn't true.

"It was just like a pure business thing," Keith says. "There was no way they were going to risk this drug taking longer to get to market. He was saying that sometimes these drugs, to push it all the way through it can cost like a billion dollars. And so any small percentage increase in that is a pretty large sum. And then you add in the fact that the really promising drugs, you're kind of racing each other to get approved first."

Keith never learned his new friend's name, but sadly, in the end, his secret source was right. Merck turned down Keith and Mikaela's requests.

She died on April 24, 2014.

*Less than five months later*, on September 4, 2014, the FDA approved the drug she had been seeking—a huge financial boon for Merck. "I think we are watching a revolutionary change in cancer therapy," Merck's head of research and development, Roger Perlmutter, declared. "Certainly the most important advance in my lifetime and maybe the most important advance since the introduction of radiotherapy."[4]

The government's stamp of approval came just a few months too late for Mikaela Knapp.

Unfortunately, she is not alone. Countless others have lost their struggle to gain access to life-saving drugs because drug companies had no incentive to provide the drugs they needed outside of clinical trials.

One of the most famous cases was that of Kianna Karnes.

Kianna was a forty-one-year-old mother of four children when she was diagnosed in 2002 with kidney cancer. She was treated with interleukin-2, the only medication approved by the FDA at the time to treat her disease. The drug nearly killed her. When that treatment failed, her father, John Rowe, began researching investigational medications.

Rowe himself was a cancer survivor, whose life had been saved because he was able to obtain a cutting-edge cancer drug, Gleevec, in a clinical trial. As a result, he had experience with the clinical trial process and how to get access to emerging medicines.

After doing some digging, he learned that both Bayer and Pfizer were conducting clinical trials for new investigational medications to treat kidney cancer—BAY 43-9006 at Bayer and SU11248 at Pfizer. But his hopes were soon dashed. Kianna was ineligible for the clinical trials because her cancer—like Mikaela Knapp's—had spread to her brain. Although surgeons had removed her brain tumors, she was still disqualified from joining the clinical trials.

So her father decided to try to get the drugs for his daughter under the FDA's expanded access program. Working with Frank Burroughs of the Abigail Alliance, he contacted Pfizer and Bayer to ask for the drug on a compassionate use basis. He got nowhere.

Rowe had worked for US congressman Dan Burton, who was then the chairman of the powerful House Government Reform Committee. As Kianna's condition deteriorated, he finally asked Congressman Burton for help. Soon, the *Wall Street Journal* took up Kianna's cause, publishing an editorial drawing attention to her plight. He told the *Journal*, "If the only alternative is death, then for God's sake let 'em have the drug." The *Journal* asked, "Who could disagree?" and called on Congress to pass a "Kianna's Law" mandating access to experimental medicines for dying patients.[5]

The public shaming and political pressure worked. The editorial appeared on March 24, 2005. That morning, the FDA told Congressman Burton's office it would approve compassionate use for Kianna. That afternoon, both companies contacted Kianna's doctor offering to make the drug available.

But sadly, it was too, little too late. Kianna died that same night at 9:41 p.m.

*Less than a year later*, both drugs were approved by the FDA. Speaking after his daughter's death, Rowe said, "I don't know that either of these drugs would have saved Kianna's life, but wouldn't it be nice to give her a chance?"

Kianna actually had a better chance than most patients at receiving expanded access. As her father explained to the *New Yorker*, "Here is a case where her old man understood clinical trials. I knew about compassionate use; I had a friendship with a powerful member of Congress; I've got the *Wall Street Journal* behind me. But I still couldn't save her life.

"Now, what about the thousands of people out there who don't have these kinds of resources available to them?" he asked.[6]

What about their right to try?

ONE EXCHANGE DURING A hearing on Right to Try in the Colorado legislature highlights why compassionate use isn't sufficient and why we need the Right to Try.

Josh Gordon, a senior research specialist with Kaiser Permanente, was testifying against Right to Try, explaining that the law was not needed.

"There is already a process in place for that through the FDA," Gordon told the committee. "It has a variety of names—compassionate use, single patient use, expanded access," he said, adding, "At Kaiser, we do have a pathway. We use the FDA's IND pathway to get access to drugs before they are approved for certain patients."

So, he was asked, how many patients got compassionate use at Kaiser Permanente?

"We typically do about four to eight single patient use requests per year," Gordon testified.

Four to eight? Millions of Americans are dying of terminal illnesses and Kaiser Permanente makes only four to eight compassionate use requests every year?

"I agree with the concept of streamlining that process," Gordon told the committee.[7]

Little wonder Right to Try passed unanimously in Colorado.

The compassionate use process needs more than just streamlining: it needs a dramatic overhaul. The FDA boasts that it approves more than 99 percent of all compassionate use requests. That sounds good, but let's take a closer look at the data.[8]

- In 2014 the FDA received 1,882 requests for expanded access and allowed 1,873 (or 99.5 percent) to proceed.
- In 2013 the agency received 977 requests, and approved 974 (99.7 percent approved).
- In 2012 the number of requests was 940 and the number approved was 936 (99.6 percent approved).
- In 2011 there were 1,200 requests and 1,199 approvals (99.9 percent approved).
- In 2010 there were 1,030 requests and 1,014 approvals (98.4 percent approved).

That is an average of twelve hundred requests each year.

So what stands out about those numbers? The FDA points to the high approval rates. But what is really striking is the infinitesimally small number of requests.

According to the American Cancer Society, in 2015 about 1,658,370 Americans will be diagnosed with cancer and 589,430 will die of it.[9] That is about 1,615 people dying of cancer *every single day*. Yet the FDA receives only twelve hundred requests for compassionate use of investigational drugs in *an entire year*?

The FDA objects that some of those requests are for multiple patients. And, it says, some people die while pursuing standard treatments, while still others may decide that, after running out of approved options, they want to stop fighting and enjoy whatever time they have left with loved ones.

Fair enough.

So how many cancer patients want access to emerging medicines but can't get them? According to the Center for Information and Study on Clinical Research Participation (CISCRP), 40 percent of all cancer patients attempt to join a clinical trial. But only 3 percent of adult cancer patients actually succeed in getting into a trial.[10]

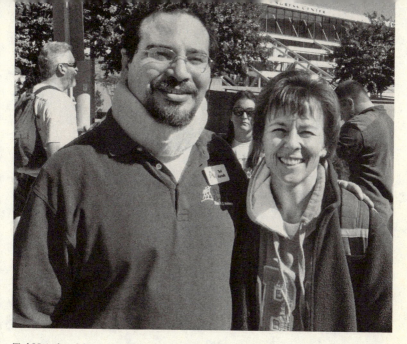

Ted Harada celebrates his miraculous recovery from ALS by completing Atlanta's two-and-a-half mile "Walk to Defeat ALS." Ted is one of just thirty-two Americans allowed to try the experimental ALS therapy. Some others in the trial saw the progression of the disease slowed or maintained the same level of functionality they had had years before the procedure. (*Courtesy of the Harada family*)

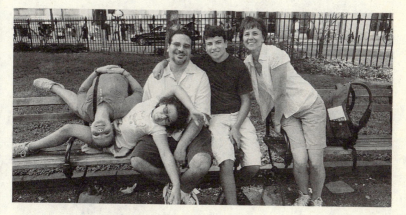

"Right now I don't need another treatment," said Ted. "But what happens when I do? If I have a treatment that's helped me twice, why should I have to go hat in hand to the FDA asking for their permission?" Under current FDA guidelines, Ted cannot undergo the procedure again. (*Courtesy of the Harada family*)

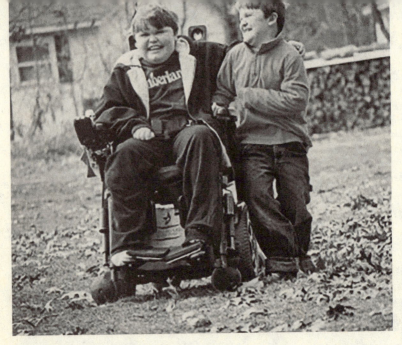

Austin and Max, Jenn McNary's sons, were both diagnosed with a deadly form of Duchenne muscular dystrophy. Max received access to a clinical trail, and Austin, Max's older brother, watched as Max's condition improved, while Austin's only got worse. (*Courtesy of Justin Ferland*)

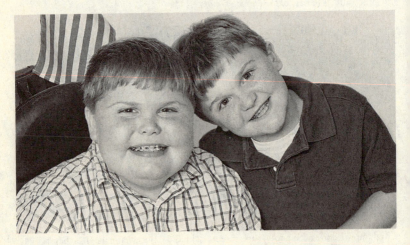

"It is one thing if your child is dying from an untreatable disease," said Jenn McNary, the boys' mother. "But to have your child dying from a treatable disease is devastating. I never thought it would be the government I was working against." (*Courtesy of Justin Ferland*)

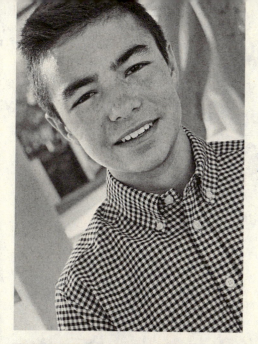

Fourteen-year-old Diego Morris and his family had to travel five thousand miles overseas to combat osteosarcoma, a deadly form of bone cancer. The lifesaving treatment Diego received is still not approved in the United States. (*Courtesy of the Goldwater Institute*)

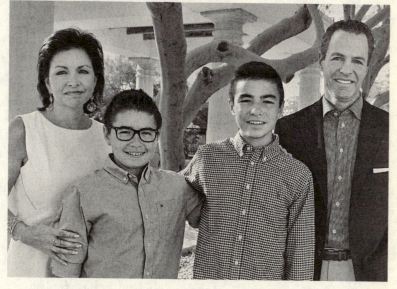

"We tried everything," said Paulina Morris, Diego's mother. "We talked to the drug manufacturer, political representatives, and the FDA. We tried every avenue to get the drug here. We realized that if we were going to get this drug for Diego, we would have to move to a foreign country." (*Courtesy of the Goldwater Institute*)

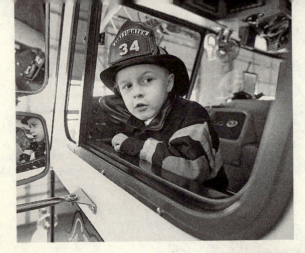

Jordan McLinn, a five-year-old with Duchenne muscular dystrophy, was granted his wish to become a fireman, then rallied fellow firefighters and legislators to pass the Right to Try law in Indiana. (*Courtesy of Chris Bergin Photography*)

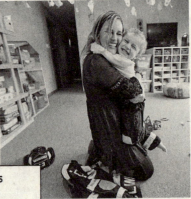

"I believe God gives us miracles in many different ways," said Laura McLinn, Jordan's mother. "He is helping people and giving people hope at just six years old. We pray that something, anything, comes through for Jordan." (*Courtesy of Chris Bergin Photography*)

---

### Jordan Joseph Nelson McLinn, Age 5
Date of Birth 5/15/09
6131 S. Meridian St. Indianapolis, IN 46217
Mommy's contact info: mslauraflowers@yahoo.com (317) 753-1661

---

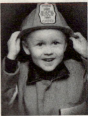

**Objective**: To obtain a job at the fire station helping the firefighters.

**Qualifications**: I am strong. I love God. I love helping people. I am super smart.

**Challenges**: I have Duchenne Muscular Dystrophy. Science says within 3 to 7 years I will be in a wheelchair and within 15 years I will most likely be living in heaven because all my muscles will be deteriorated. We don't really believe that though.

**Skills**: Taking Care of Dogs, Cleaning, Building Things, Playing with Cars & Trucks, Dancing, Cooking, Making People Smile

---

*Jordan says he wants to be a firefighter when he grows up. He was given a fatal diagnosis of DMD last year. It would be awesome if there is anything he can do maybe once a week for a short time to help out at the fire station. We are pretty flexible with days/times. He is an awesome little boy, happy and full of life! Please let me know if I can bring him in for an "interview". Thank you for your consideration.*

*- Laura McLinn ©*

To bring joy to Jordan and raise awareness for Duchenne, Laura McLinn posted her son's résumé to Facebook. Within hours, Jordan received job offers from fire stations all across the country. (*Courtesy of the McLinn Family*)

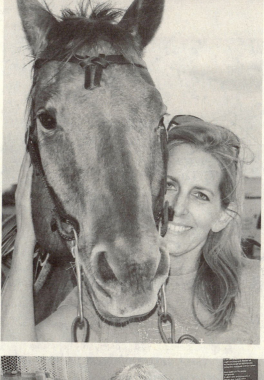

Andrea Sloan of Texas, unable to qualify for a clinical trial, sought "compassionate use" access to BMN-673, an experimental cancer drug. Despite widespread public support, the drug manufacturer BioMarin refused to engage in a dialogue or even to look at her medical records. (*Courtesy of the Sloan family*)

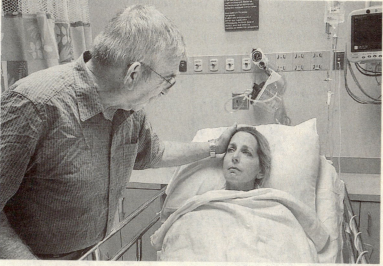

FDA approval was too little too late. "Andrea's scans showed the drug was having incredible success," said Karen Sloan, Andrea's mother. "But the months of trying to engage BioMarin had taken its toll; the pneumonia proved insurmountable to her physical body." Andrea passed away on New Year's Day 2014. (*Courtesy of the Sloan family*)

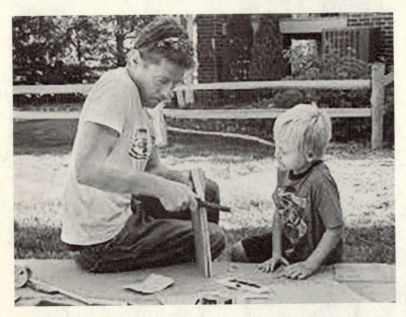

Nick Audin petitioned for and was denied access to PD-1, a potentially lifesaving experimental drug. Nick's wife, Amy, launched SaveLockysDad.com, a website with a moving video featuring Nick's towheaded seven-year-old son, Lachlan "Locky" Audin. (*Courtesy of the Auden family*)

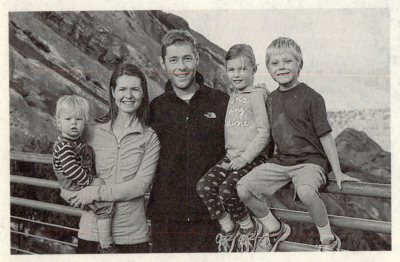

"We needed hope but didn't receive it through our battle," said Amy. "For the patients and for their families, Right to Try offers some hope." (*Courtesy of the Auden family*)

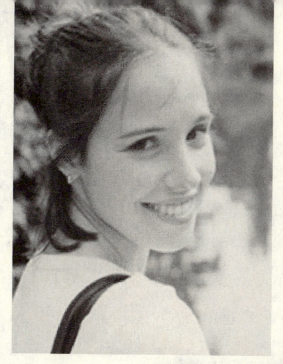

Abigail Burroughs's inability to gain access to the investigational cancer drug Eribitux may have contributed to her death. Abigail's father, Frank, formed Abigail Alliance, then sued the FDA to help others like Abigail get the lifesaving drugs they need. (*Courtesy of Frank Burroughs*)

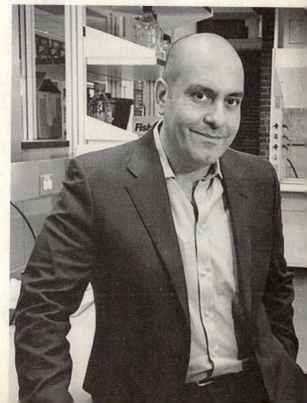

Chris Garabedian resigned his position as CEO of Sarepta after struggles with the FDA. "Once a drug moves forward, and it's successful, everybody forgets about the delays, the inefficiency of the process, what boys [with Duchenne] could have been helped if this were approved a year ago." (*Courtesy of Chris Garabedian*)

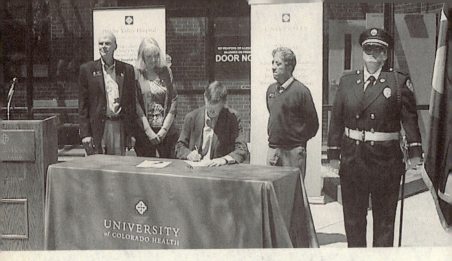

Colorado becomes the first state in the nation to sign Right to Try into law when governor John Hickenlooper signs House Bill 1282, sending a strong message to Washington. Republicans and Democrats agree on little these days, but there is unanimity in Colorado when it comes to defending the Right to Try. (*Courtesy of KCNC-TV Denver*)

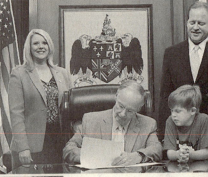

Governor Robert Bentley signs Senate Bill 357, the Gabe's Right to Try Act, into law. The bill was inspired by ten-year-old Gabe Griffin, who has Duchenne muscular dystrophy. (*Courtesy of the State of Alabama Governor's Office*)

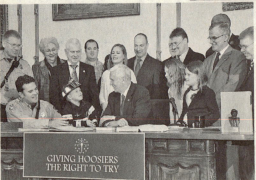

Five-year-old honorary fireman Jordan McLinn, the McLinn family, and local firemen from IFD Station 13 look on as Indiana governor Mike Pence signs the Right to Try bill into law. (*Courtesy of the Indiana State Republican Caucus*)

Why is that? As Dr. Emil Freireich, the MD Anderson Cancer Center doctor who pioneered the cure for childhood acute lymphoblastic leukemia, explains in the *British Medical Journal*, "most cancer patients cannot participate in phase II trials because they are either ineligible or they are unable to fulfill the financial and social requirements for participating in such trials, such as staying in the centers conducting these trials, sometimes for many weeks or months." Moreover, Dr. Freireich says, in many cases trials "are designed to give the highest probability of a positive outcome. Thus, they have patient eligibility requirements which assure that only the healthiest patients at the earliest point in their disease are entered. These decisions are not based on any reasonable evidence that patients who are ineligible would not benefit, but are strictly designed to fulfil the regulatory requirements established by bodies such as the Federal [Food and] Drug Administration (FDA) and the regulatory components of industry and academia that govern these clinical trials."[11]

And the problem is getting worse. According to the Tufts Center for the Study of Drug Development, the total number of eligibility criteria for clinical trials has nearly doubled over the past decade, making it harder and harder for patients to qualify.[12]

If 40 percent of cancer patients try to get into trials and only 3 percent succeed, that means most fail to get access to emerging treatments through clinical trials. Since there will be about 1,658,370 new cancer diagnoses in 2015, that means there are hundreds of thousands of cancer patients who want experimental medicines but cannot get them. And that is not counting all the hundreds of thousands of other Americans who will be diagnosed with other terminal illnesses this year.

And yet the FDA considers twelve hundred compassionate use requests each year a system that "seems to work quite well"?

When so many Americans are fighting terminal illnesses and fewer than 1 percent are getting access to investigational drugs, the system isn't working well. It is broken. Either patients don't know that they can apply for investigational treatments through compassionate use, or the barriers to applying are so overwhelming that patients and doctors cannot overcome them, or they don't bother to try.

In all likelihood, the answer is all of the above. Keith and Mikaela Knapp's first doctor did not even tell them compassionate use was an option. It was only because they were lucky enough to find another doctor who told them about compassionate use (and was willing to fill out a hundred hours of paperwork) that they learned they could pursue an experimental treatment.

Many doctors simply can't spend the time it takes to get access to emerging drugs, especially when it means taking weeks off from treating other patients. One doctor at a leading cancer hospital told me that he had never once applied for compassionate use for a patient. "It's just too daunting," he said.

For many doctors, a patient getting compassionate access is like the mythical unicorn—a creature that legends say exists, but one no one has actually ever seen. Earlier, we met Andrea Sloan—the Texas lawyer who died after a long battle trying to get access to an experimental drug. Her oncologist at MD Anderson Cancer Center, Dr. Charles Levenback, told CBS News, "I cannot recall in my practice in the last 10 years a patient who got compassionate use of a drug."[13]

Think about that: when compassionate use is so rare that a leading cancer specialist at one of the nation's leading cancer research hospitals has never seen it happen in the last ten years, there is clearly something deeply wrong with the system.

As his MD Anderson colleague Dr. Freireich explains, "It is tragic that regulatory bodies have created a circumstance where people have to live in an aura of hopelessness even though they have the will, the resources, and the ability to expose themselves to the risk of participating in investigational studies and to enjoy the potential for benefit.

The solution is legislation or judicial action to permit expanded access to experimental treatments for patients with limited life expectancy.

"Patients with advanced cancer and limited life expectancy should have the same privilege as all individuals in a free society—that is, to decide their own benefit [to] risk ratio," he says.[14]

The vast majority of doctors agree. In 2015 SERMO, a social network for medical doctors, asked 2,182 physicians, "Should compassionate use be allowed for unproven drugs or therapies?" An overwhelming 93 percent of the doctors said yes, while only 7 percent were opposed.[15]

Polls also show that doctors see the FDA as an obstacle to their ability to get cutting-edge treatments for their patients. For many years the Competitive Enterprise Institute has polled medical specialists about their attitudes toward the FDA—orthopedic surgeons (2007), oncologists (2002), emergency room doctors (1999), neurologists and neurosurgeons (1998), and cardiologists (1996).[16] And over the years, the institute has found the same consistent results: by wide margins, these specialty doctors—those most likely to treat terminally ill patients—believe that (1) the FDA takes too long to approve drugs, (2) the FDA hinders their ability to treat patients, and (3) patients should have much broader access to investigational drugs and medical devices that have not yet been approved by the FDA.

- When asked, "Would you say the FDA's approval process has hurt your ability to treat your patients with the best possible care?" 80 percent of neurologists and neurosurgeons said yes, as did 78 percent of orthopedic surgeons, 77 percent of oncologists, 71 percent of cardiologists, and 58 percent of emergency room doctors.
- When asked, "Do you agree or disagree with the following statement: the FDA is too slow in approving new drugs and medical devices?" 76 percent of orthopedic surgeons agreed, along with 67 percent of neurologists and neurosurgeons, 65

percent of cardiologists, 64 percent of emergency room doctors, and 61 percent of oncologists.

- When asked whether they would support a "proposal to change FDA law so that unapproved drugs or medical devices could be made available to physicians as long as they carried a warning label about their unapproved status," 73 percent of neurologists and neurosurgeons said they would, as did 70 percent of orthopedic surgeons, 69 percent of emergency room doctors, and 68 percent of oncologists.

In other words, the vast majority of doctors believe that people who are fighting for their lives have a right to try investigational treatments. Yet it is not happening—at least not on a scale that remotely meets the needs of patients and the desires of their treating physicians.

So who is to blame for this sad state of affairs?

The drug companies blame the FDA.

They believe that if their emerging drugs are taken by the sickest patients, like Mikaela, who have exhausted their standard treatments, these patients will have a higher incidence of mortality and their drugs will appear less promising. These "less promising" results could cause the FDA to require years more testing and cost millions of dollars—a risk that companies don't want to take.

In 2010 the Biotechnology Industry Organization issued a white paper outlining the "dilemma" its member companies face when they receive compassionate use requests.[17] When patients ask for compassionate access, they wrote, "biotech companies must balance those interests with their responsibility to move products through the regulatory process to receive marketing approval; a process that could be delayed or put at risk by providing access to the product outside of a clinical trial."

They listed two principal risks companies face from FDA regulators.

First, they cited the risk that compassionate access could cause the FDA to delay approval of their new drugs:

Since the company will be providing an unapproved product to a patient outside the scope of a clinical trial . . . should an adverse event occur with a patient in the early access program, the company puts its broader clinical testing program at risk since the FDA may require the company to initiate new clinical trials or expand existing trials as part of its investigation of the event. This could delay or even prevent the approval of the product. Consequently, a larger patient population may be denied a potentially beneficial product.

In some circumstances, therefore, by allowing early access, the company risks market approval of the product. Thus, the question often confronting companies is whether to put an entire project at risk—and therefore jeopardize availability of a drug for a larger patient population—in order to provide early access to a product for an individual or small group of patients.

Second, the Biotech Industry Organization says, if compassionate use becomes widespread, it will be harder to recruit patients for the large, randomized placebo trials that the FDA requires (in which some patients receive the drug while others get sugar water):

If patients knew they could access a treatment outside the clinical trial process, it would reduce their incentive to enroll in a trial especially since they may receive a placebo and therefore not be treated for their illness. Therefore, if early access programs become extremely common, the clinical trials system could break down, delaying or ending some product development programs.

More recently, two Merck executives—Michael Rosenblatt and Bruce Kuhlik—wrote in the May 2015 issue of *JAMA: The Journal of the American Medical Association* that expanded access programs (EAPs) pose real risks: conduct of an EAP may jeopardize enrollment or retention of patients in ongoing clinical trials of a drug that determine safety and efficacy and ultimately gain regulatory approval. . . . Because many patients requesting early access are extremely ill and are outside the profile of patients eligible to participate in clinical trials, serious adverse events, including death, occur. If such an event occurs in an EAP, it might not be possible to determine if it is drug-related. As a result, a promising therapy might be delayed, or even abandoned before sufficient clinical trial data can be generated.[18]

Asked about these concerns, Dr. Janet Woodcock, director of the FDA's Center for Drug Evaluation and Research, insisted that the FDA is not a deterrent to compassionate use. "We serve the people that take medicine: the patients, the people who need medicine. That's the reason we're here and that's what we do, that's our mission," she said in an interview. "We serve them by trying to get drugs that are reasonably well studied on the market as expeditiously as possible, evaluating those drugs while they're on the market to make sure that nothing untoward happens. And also we do believe and do run a lot of access programs obviously because we think people should have the ability to take an investigational drug if they don't have other alternatives. That's what we think.

"There are a lot of problems with this, so we acknowledge those," she says. But she adds, "We don't usually stand in the way of access. It's up to the companies whether or not they provide these programs and at what level. And they can publicize them and make them widely available, or they can only respond to calls, or they can refuse to have an access program."

What does she make of industry's concern that granting compassionate access could cause the FDA to delay drug approvals?

"Well, they certainly say that," Dr. Woodcock says. "We've heard that hundreds of times. We know of only one instance where we took some action based on what we observed—and that was pretty recent actually—in an access program. So we don't think [that is a legitimate reason]."

She says she understands that companies fear the FDA. "Well, we hold sort of the power of whether they're going to be successful with their development program or not. People are afraid of the IRS too. Regulators are not popular. It's not our 'job' really," she says. "There's a huge amount of risk in drug development because there's so many failures. They want to be conservative, but we don't think that's a very valid excuse."

She says that the drug companies, not the FDA, are the main obstacle to expanding access to emerging drugs. "We don't, as I said, stand between patients who are dying getting access to investigational drugs. But I get that the companies don't always want to run access programs."

If it is not fear of jeopardizing FDA approval or clinical trials, then what is the reason?

"I think there are a lot of reasons that companies don't want to give drugs out," she says. "It's a very expensive thing to run an access program."

Is it FDA's responsibility to help patients get access to experimental treatments?

"To the extent we are capable of," Dr. Woodcock says. She says the FDA has a twenty-four-hour call line for emergency requests. "Our doctors and our other personnel are often arranging access." And she says the agency is working on establishing a clearinghouse that will provide "one-stop shopping" for doctors seeking approval for access requests. "We have talked to [members of Congress] and we had a meeting with some patient advocates a few months ago . . . and talked about could the companies post their policies, number one; and then could there be established some kind of clearinghouse so there would be one-stop shopping. . . . Somebody to call if you wanted access to an experimental drug and then hopefully they could work those things out."

But, she says, there is only so much the FDA can do.

"We do not make or develop the drugs. We don't own the drugs," she says. "We can't extract drugs out of the hands of companies and give them to people."

So here is where it stands: The drug companies blame the FDA. The FDA blames the drug companies. Meanwhile, patients are dying—and no one is doing much of anything to help patients access promising drugs and treatments.

So what is the solution?

First, we need to create grassroots pressure for change. That is what the Right to Try movement is doing. Today, the FDA touts its expanded access program as a reason why Right to Try is unnecessary. But back in the 1980s, when AIDS activists chained themselves to the gates of the FDA demanding expanded access, the FDA said *that program* was unnecessary too—often using virtually the same language it uses against Right to Try.

In February 1988 FDA commissioner Frank Young declared, "We've been working very rapidly in getting new drugs into people," adding that the "FDA is not the bottleneck"[19] and "the real hang-up is the science."[20] At the FDA, he said, "We feel it's important that people have access to drugs as soon as possible."[21] To do that, FDA spokesman Don McClaren said, "We have to balance [dying patients' concerns] with the legal requirement that the drugs we license are safe and effective."[22]

If that sounds familiar, it's because FDA officials are singing the same tune today. "I don't think we are a barrier to access for patients,"[23] FDA commissioner Margaret Hamburg declared in 2014, but "at the end of the day we have to be guided by science in everything we do. It has to be our compass."[24] She added that "we adapt and improve models and timetables to help patients get earlier access to promising new drugs," but said that "we must balance the eagerness to find ways to get promising treatments to patients as quickly as possible . . . with the need to provide assurance that the benefits of these treatments outweigh the risks."[25]

The officials are still deploying the same, worn-out arguments thirty years later.

In 1980 AIDS activists rejected the FDA's claim that everything was fine, and demanded fundamental reform. "[The advocacy group] ACT UP's fundamental contention was that, with a new epidemic disease such as AIDS, testing experimental new therapies is itself a form of health care and that access to health care must be everyone's right," wrote Douglas Crimp, an activist.[26] Not only did activists protest; they exercised their Right to Try by organizing networks of underground pharmacies, or "buyers clubs," that distributed unapproved drugs, often imported from overseas, to dying members of the AIDS community.[27]

These were acts of civil disobedience, and they put lifesaving drugs in the hands of the dying. They shamed the FDA into changing its policies, saved lives, and gave birth to our compassionate use system.

Today, as we have seen, that system is not meeting the needs of dying patients, who are still not getting access to the drugs they need. So the Right to Try movement is picking up the mantle and continuing the fight for change.

Instead of using underground pharmacies, the Right to Try movement is using state law to expand access to emerging drugs. Instead of chaining ourselves to the gates of the FDA, we are harnessing the power of millions of Americans to get our message to Washington: Compassionate use is broken, and Americans with terminal illnesses don't have time to wait.

The Right to Try movement is using state constitutions exactly as our Founding Fathers intended—as "instrument[s] of redress"

(Alexander Hamilton, *Federalist* number 28). We are using the states to reclaim our fundamental rights and pressure the federal government to change course.

And that pressure is starting to work.

For years doctors have been complaining about the FDA's application forms for compassionate access, which even by the agency's admission take over a hundred hours to fill out. It is daunting even for doctors from major research hospitals, who are used to filling out mountains of paperwork for clinical trials. But for a local community doctor seeking compassionate access for a single patient, getting FDA approval is like climbing Mount Kilimanjaro. One hundred hours is two and a half weeks of working full-time doing nothing but filling out government paperwork. Few doctors can afford that kind of time. As a result, few seek compassionate use of investigational medicines for their patients—one reason why the FDA receives so few applications.

In May 2014 FDA commissioner Margaret Hamburg appeared on NPR's *Diane Rehm Show*, where she said that "in numerous cases we have proceeded within 24 hours or overnight. We move these applications as expeditiously as possible." And she expressed shock that other guests had suggested the application process for compassionate use was too complicated. "I was surprised . . . to hear about how cumbersome the process is and how it takes weeks or months at the FDA," she said. "I'm looking at the form now. It's three pages long. A lot of it is checking off boxes."[28]

But on February 4, 2015—nine months after Commissioner Hamburg claimed getting compassionate use was a simple as "checking off boxes"—the FDA suddenly did an about-face.

Writing on the FDA's blog, associate commissioner Dr. Peter Lurie declared, "We heard concerns from patients and physicians that the process for gaining access to investigational drugs was too difficult, and pulled together a team to find a way to make that process simpler."

After reviewing the forms, Dr. Lurie wrote, FDA officials concluded that "the existing application form was too complex: it called for 26 separate types of information and seven attachments. In fact, it was originally designed for manufacturers seeking to begin human testing, not for physicians seeking use by single patients."

He announced that the FDA had created a new form that would be much easier for physicians to use. "We estimate that physicians will be able to complete the finalized version of the [new] form in just 45 minutes, as compared to the 100 hours listed on the previous form," he wrote. "Additionally, to further assist the physician seeking access to an experimental therapy, we have redesigned our website to make it easier to navigate and to explain the new proposed process in detail."[29]

For Frank Burroughs of the Abigail Alliance, the announcement was vindication.

"We were right!" he says. "It took too long!"

In an interview, Dr. Woodcock proudly touted this reform. "We have streamlined the process, which was excessively onerous."

But just a few months earlier, her then-boss, FDA Commissioner Hamburg, said it wasn't "onerous" at all—just a matter of "checking off boxes."

What suddenly changed?

Here is what changed: by February 2015, five state legislatures had passed Right to Try laws eliminating the need for the FDA's compassionate use program. Only in the face of this grassroots revolt did the FDA finally acknowledge what doctors and patients had been saying for years: that the forms were too difficult and the process was too complex. Only after states started passing Right to Try laws did the FDA finally admit, after repeated public denials, that the application did in fact, take one hundred hours.

At this writing, the new, shorter application *still* has not yet been put into effect. An FDA spokesman says, "We're hoping to have it launched by the end of the year." But even if it is eventually put in place, a simplified form is only an incremental step forward.

It does not solve the fundamental problem: you still have to beg the federal government for the Right to Try to save your own life.

The problem is not just a hundred hours of paperwork; it is an entire system of federal disincentives that block and discourage access to investigational medicines. Without deeper reforms, simplified paperwork will be nothing more than window dressing for an inhumane system that prevents hundreds of thousands of dying Americans from getting the drugs they need to survive.

If just five states passing Right to Try laws can force the FDA to eliminate ninety-nine hours of paperwork, imagine what can be accomplished when Right to Try is the law of the land in all fifty states. We need to keep up the pressure until compassionate access is the rule for everyone facing a terminal illness, not the exception for a privileged few.

And that requires not only removing the bureaucratic obstacles that discourage doctors from applying for compassionate use but also getting rid of the bureaucratic obstacles that discourage companies from making their drugs available to desperate patients.

When we speak with CEOs of biotech and pharmaceutical companies, the two biggest risks they cite in regard to expanding compassionate access are that it will (1) delay drug approvals and (2) drive patients out of clinical trials.

Both of these problems can be solved—but it will require changing the way the FDA does business.

If we want companies to dramatically increase compassionate use, they must have confidence that granting access to experimental treatments is not going to delay the approval of drugs and cost them millions of dollars in lost business.

Today, that is not the case. As one biotech CEO told me, "Sponsors generally believe that the FDA puts the burden of proof on the company to convince the regulatory reviewers that any adverse event is not related to the company's drug. While there may not be a lot of examples that suggest that adverse events uncovered in a compassionate use/ expanded access situation [have] derailed a drug, it is one of the reasons that it has not been more widely adopted because of the theoretical risk that such adverse events will constitute a disproportionate amount of attention in the dialogue with regulatory reviewers in the effort to get a drug approved."

Former FDA commissioner Andy von Eschenbach (who supports dramatically increasing compassionate use through federal, not state-level, reforms) says that today "there's no upside for the company other than doing a moral good. But there is an awful lot of downside for them."

For some, simply doing a moral good is incentive enough. One CEO of a major pharmaceutical company says it already does make its drugs available on a compassionate basis. "I think it's really important that promising new drugs get to patients sooner. I've worked all my life with that goal, not only in the US, but around the world."

This CEO says that while "we certainly, in our programs, have found ways to address that compassionate need," there is a fear among others in the industry that "if you use your product in really sick people, the illness the person has may be interpreted as side effects of the drug. That's what people are worried about in many instances."

To address this concern, the FDA needs to create "safe harbor" for drug companies that provide their products to patients outside clinical trials, and make clear it will hold companies harmless in the regulatory process if they do the right thing and provide drugs for dying patients.

You can't just ignore the data if a patient dies, says Dr. von Eschenbach, but you can find "a way to *sequester* the data. . . . In other words, it certainly has to be recorded and recognized. [But you] find a way to recognize the data but also recognize the circumstance and not allow it to inappropriately adversely influence the regulatory decision."

The FDA was supposed to make its policies on sequestration clear in 2009, when the agency last updated its compassionate access programs. But according to the pharmaceutical industry, it still has not done so. Speaking on NPR's *Diane Rehm Show* in May 2014, Sascha Haverfield, the vice president for scientific and regulatory affairs at the Pharmaceutical Research and Manufacturers of America (PhRMA), said, "You want to provide certainty to the process to drug developers to understand how data will be used. . . . When the FDA put this process in place in 2009, we are still looking for final guidance on how FDA will facilitate the process and use data."[30]

Five years later, at the time of this writing, the FDA has still not provided clear guidance to companies on how it will treat data from compassionate use. No wonder companies are reluctant to provide access.

Dr. Woodcock says the FDA is still working on it. "We are completely aware [of those concerns] and we're working on sort of a statement that we get to say that we don't hold these experiences against the drug."

How many states will have to pass Right to Try laws before the FDA finally gets around to issuing it?

Sequestration is important, but it's only the first step. If we want to dramatically increase the scope and scale of compassionate use, we also need to create *incentives* for companies to cooperate with compassionate use requests.

"Making it easier is getting rid of the drag," Dr. von Eschenbach says. But the bigger question is, "How do you do the pull? Is there a positive way of incentivizing it? There's got to be a positive incentive as well as getting rid of the barriers."

One incentive he proposes is to reward drug companies that offer drugs on an "off-label" basis before FDA approval. Today, patients are regularly rejected for clinical trials because they have the "right" kind of cancer in the "wrong" part of the body. This is what happened to Mikaela Knapp and Abigail Burroughs. They did not qualify for trials, because of the location of their cancer, even though the drugs they needed were the right ones to treat the type of cancer they had.

Sadly, Dr. von Eschenbach says, this happens all the time. He explains that a drug manufacturer may be conducting clinical trials on a promising new drug for, say, lung cancer, when it is approached by a patient with pancreatic cancer who does not qualify for the clinical trial. But it turns out the pancreatic tumor has the same genetic mutation that is apparently driving the lung cancer in the manufacturer's clinical trial.

If the drug were already approved, doctors would simply go ahead and use the lung cancer drug to treat pancreatic cancer—no special FDA permission would be required. This is called using a drug off-label—because the FDA label says the drug is for lung cancer, but the doctor is confident it can work in pancreatic cancer as well. "Oncology was built on off-label use," Dr. von Eschenbach says. "What happens all the time with that scenario is, if the drug's already available, then it's simply used off-label and everybody's happy as a clam."

He believes we should do the same thing "in the very, very early stages of clinical development, before a drug has been approved and [is] available on the market and everyone can get access to it by prescription."

This can be done by (1) promising to sequester the data from the pancreatic patient, so that it does not hurt the lung-cancer trial if something goes wrong and (2) promising that if the drug works, positive data will be collected and could be used to help the company win approval from the FDA to market the drug for pancreatic as well as lung cancer—which is very financially valuable for the company.

"If it pans out that that drug is active in that pancreatic patient, they're one step further along in developing another indication for their drug," he says. "Rather than having to go all the way back to square one and doing another full-blown registration study for a completely different indication, you have sort of a shortcut and you can get an additional label indication with a minimal amount of required data. . . . And then if a sufficient number of patients get access to the drug earlier, you take that back to the FDA and use it as a registry.

"If it doesn't work," he says, "the data's recorded and recognized but it's not going to count against the lung-cancer registry protocol."

Now, suddenly, compassionate use is a win-win for industry. The company now has an economic reason, as well as a moral reason, to provide access.

This "could get the companies and the sponsors to be much more liberal about their willingness to provide these drugs," Dr. von Eschenbach says. But to make it happen "you really have to incentivize the sponsor by protecting them and giving them an opportunity to advance their goal of drug development."

Some companies already do this, even in the face of regulatory obstacles. One CEO of a major pharmaceutical company described to me how his company many years ago offered a drug on a compassionate use basis to patients on a transplant list.

"We thought we could let them live longer until they could find an [organ]," he says, "but they in fact came off of the transplant list. Their disease regressed." His company had no idea its drug would be so effective in patients with advanced disease until it offered the drug to them under compassionate use.

We need to find ways to encourage more companies to take those kinds of risks. We need policies that reward companies for doing the right thing, and change early access from a "dilemma" for industry into a tool of scientific discovery.

The second big obstacle that drug companies cite is the risk that expanding compassionate use will discourage patients from joining clinical trials. The problem here, once again, is caused by the FDA and its overreliance on what are called "double-blind placebo controlled trials"—studies in which some patients get the experimental medicine and others do not.

As Steven Walker, cofounder of the Abigail Alliance, points out, the problem is "the FDA's retention of obsolete clinical trial designs, in which terminal and seriously ill patients must be coerced to enroll in agency-required trials under the risk of randomization to a placebo, or an older, known to be inadequate drug, as the basis of its entire regulatory scheme."[31]

He says, "Enrolling in a randomized placebo control trial is far more dangerous to a patient with a terminal disease than it would be to simply be given the drug. Because getting the placebo, under blinded conditions, is for many, many people a death sentence. It's a gamble. The company is betting that fewer people will die in the arm that gets the drug than in the placebo arm. This pile of bodies is smaller than the placebo pile, that's what they want to see. And that's literally what they are measuring. That is our clinical research system for cancer."[32]

The excruciating dilemma these studies create for patients and their families was recently brought to life in the Ken Burns documentary *Cancer: The Emperor of All Maladies*.

In one scene, the parents of a leukemia-stricken fourteen-month-old girl named Olivia Blair are discussing with her doctors whether to enroll her in a clinical trial for a new chemotherapy drug.

"This is probably the hardest decision along the way that you guys have to make," a doctor tells Olivia's parents.

Her mom, Kelly, leans across the table and asks, almost in a whisper, "So how do we find out if they get the [drug]? How do we find that out? It's randomized, right?"

The doctor explains how the selection process work. Names of patients are put into a computer that decides who gets the drug and who doesn't. "There's a formula that spits out, 'OK, the next patient that consents is going to get it, the next patient is not going to get it.'"

Kelly pauses with a confused look. "That's like . . . I don't . . . I don't . . . I don't feel comfortable with that."

The doctor tries to reassure her. "The thought of your child's treatment being left up to a computer is a very hard concept to take. It's OK if you decide not to be in the study."

"I don't know what to say," Kelly tells the doctors.

The doctors leave the room, and the family holds hands as Olivia's father, Marcus, leads them in prayer:

"Lord, what we ask of you now Father is just to kind of nudge us in the right direction, Lord, and put us at ease and at peace with the decision that is ultimately made. And we just humbly ask for your guidance in making this decision, Lord. Amen."

It is a moral outrage that any Americans with a life-threatening illness—much less the parents of a fourteen-month-old baby with cancer—should be forced by their own government to make this kind of decision.

For decades, patient advocates have been demanding that the government stop putting people facing terminal diagnoses in placebo trials. When AIDS protesters chained themselves to the gates at FDA headquarters in the 1990s, one of their key demands was:

> No more double-blind placebo trials. Because giving a placebo to someone with a life-threatening illness is unethical, the FDA must inform designers of clinical trials that it will not accept data based on placebo trials. Instead, new drugs must be measured against other approved drugs or, where there are none, against other experimental therapies, different doses of the same drug, or against what is already known of the natural progression of AIDS.[33]

They were morally right then.

But the difference today is that there is no longer any scientific justification for continuing this unethical approach to clinical trials—because technology is increasingly making these trials unnecessary.

"The reason why we have randomized placebo control trials is it's an artifact of an age when you couldn't analyze large data sets effectively and look for, and tease out, one variable from all of the things that were changing in a large data set," says Dr. Scott Gottlieb, a former FDA deputy commissioner and a scholar at the American Enterprise Institute. "But in today's age, when we have sophisticated computers that look at large data sets and tease out with high degrees of certainty statistical conclusions based on how different groups are being affected, you could be incorporating those tools into drug development. And on the medical device side they actually do, but on the drug development side they don't."

When Kianna Karnes was waging her unsuccessful campaign to get access to an experimental cancer drug, the *Wall Street Journal* pointed out:

The problem here is the FDA's unethical—and let us stress, unscientific—insistence on gathering information about drugs by way of "blinded" placebo-controlled trials, in which a subset of study patients are knowingly denied the new treatment and in some cases denied access to any active treatment at all. This may be moral with an antihistamine; it's certainly not with treatments for a terminal disease.

What's more, it's entirely unnecessary. We already know what happens to most cancer patients who don't get treated. They die. We generally know, on average, how long that will take. . . . A deadly follow-on effect of the placebo fetish is that it gives companies a disincentive to run compassionate use programs for unapproved drugs. That's because companies won't be able to satisfy FDA demands to enroll patients in placebo trials if patients know they can get the drug for sure (instead of running the risk of getting a sugar pill) through compassionate use. Hence Mrs. Karnes's deadly predicament.[34]

The time has come for the FDA to give up its placebo fetish and start relying more on open-label trials instead, trials in which all the patients are actually getting the experimental drug.

Open-label studies are more than sufficient to determine whether a drug is safe and effective. Indeed, the FDA has relied on them in the past. "A lot of breakthrough therapies were approved on the basis of open-label studies where everyone got the drug and FDA allowed you to match them against historical controls and basically discern whether there was drug effect by looking at how patients should have done relative to how they did in the trial," Dr. Gottlieb says.

But today, when technology is making placebo trials less necessary, he says, the FDA's insistence on them is growing. "Now FDA wants these really pristine, tightly randomized experiments, what I call the perfect experiment . . . clinical trial results that are so mathematically rigorous that they leave absolutely not a shred of a doubt that the magnitude of the benefit that you're observing in the clinical trial is the drug's true benefit. And because they're requiring these kinds of trials, it forecloses the opportunity to give the drug away outside the trial."

So how do we fix this problem?

All it takes, Dr. Gottlieb says, is changing one word in the law.

Right now, the FDA has all the legal authority it needs under the FDA Modernization Act to approve drugs on the basis of open-label studies. The problem is that it rarely exercises that authority.

So the answer is for Congress to take that discretion away.

"Congress should reaffirm the provisions of the Modernization Act. It should spell out in legislation that the FDA 'shall'—rather than 'may'—approve drugs for severe conditions on the basis of a single study, or a more lenient statistical orthodoxy than 'two, randomized, placebo controlled trials,'" Dr. Gottlieb says.[35] "You change a single word in the statute and you've made a tremendous amount of difference, you've taken away FDA's discretion to require these ridiculous placebo controlled trials in settings where it doesn't make sense."

Dr. von Eschenbach, the former FDA commissioner, is in complete agreement. "Scott's absolutely right. I mean, there are ways now, different technologies and methodologies that are significantly reducing our dependence on phase III blinded randomization."

The fact is that we already know that the regulatory system can function without placebo-controlled trials, because the FDA already does it—in its medical device division. As the *Wall Street Journal* put it, "Nobody gets placebo defibrillators in trials."[36] If open-label studies are the norm for medical devices, there is no reason why they can't be the norm for medicines as well.

Not only would greater reliance on open-label studies increase compassionate access; it would also help drug companies increase participation in clinical trials. If patients knew they were certain they would get the drug and not a placebo, more people would join trials. And, given the choice, most would probably choose a trial over compassionate use—because drugs are expensive and the trial is free.

So again, it is a win-win for drug companies. They get more trial participants and have an even greater incentive to grant early access as well.

Another obstacle to compassionate access is supply. When the drug in question is a small molecule pill or the sponsor is a giant pharmaceutical company, supply is usually not an issue. As one CEO put it, these products have "a simple manufacturing process where scaling up for a larger volume of patients constitutes a rounding error on overall drug development and manufacturing costs."

But for more complex drugs and biologics—especially those produced by small companies operating on shoestring budgets—the companies depend on research-stage manufacturing capacity that typically is supply constrained. Ramping up manufacturing to get more supply during the clinical development phase for compassionate use isn't possible. There simply is no way, this CEO says, to justify "the cost, resources, and risk in scaling up and preparing to offer a larger volume of drug than is needed for clinical trials prior to knowing if the drug has performed favorably in the pivotal trials."

If we want manufacturers to create more supply early in the clinical trial process, then we have to allow them to derive an economic benefit from making the drug available. The simple fact is: these are companies, and money talks. "The most potent incentive is to allow companies to charge for investigational drugs prior to approval," says Chris Garabedian, the Sarepta Therapeutics CEO whose company pioneered the Duchenne drug that saved Jenn McNary's son.

Today, federal law prohibits companies from making a profit from emerging drugs (though they can recover costs). This means early access is essentially an act of charity—one that many smaller companies on shoestring budgets can rarely afford, especially on a large scale. Allowing companies to charge for investigational drugs would make compassionate use instantly more attractive. For smaller companies operating on shoestring budgets, it might even be a way to help them finance their research and clinical trials.

Garabedian says that for-profit compassionate use models already exist. In France, for example, the government has a policy called temporary authorization for use (ATU), which allows companies to provide experimental drugs and charge for them at the expected market price or higher.[37] "The French ATU is widely used, and often the first step for a company to gain access to a market and generate revenues for providing early access," he says. "Other countries also allow reimbursement (with profit) prior to approval." But the United States does not.

Without the ability to charge for the drug, he says, no CEO could justify creating a large expanded access program to his or her investors. He points out that most drug manufacturers are public companies and that many precommercial pharmaceutical and biotech companies are not yet profitable.

"Investors in these companies have an influence on deployment of capital and the appropriate use of resources," Garabedian says. They "do not want to see unnecessary (read: cash draining activity vs. cash generating activity) initiatives without a tangible link to the market value of the company."

This means that "most CEOs would be criticized by investors and financial media, not hailed, by announcing a broad expanded access program. It would be hard to justify the cost-risk benefit of such an approach." As a result, Garabedian says, "large-scale use and adoption of early access will not occur until we . . . allow a profitable pricing model preapproval as in the case of France's ATU program."

Dr. von Eschenbach would go even further. Rather than charging for treatments, he recommends that the FDA simply allow companies to put drugs out on the market much earlier in their clinical development, with a rigorous system of "postmarket surveillance" in place. Once a drug's safety has been established, "if you allowed the drug to go out on the market when you had less than 100 percent certainty [of efficacy], but you had a really good system of post-market surveillance . . . you can continue to expand the experiential database so that you get closer and closer to certainty. . . . But you don't have to be depriving people of that until you get to that 'I'm 99 percent certain I understand how it works because I forced you to put so many people on the trial and carry it out for such a long period of time that it's obvious as the nose on the end of your face.'"

This way "people won't have to wait eight years, they can get it earlier, and it's actually approved and it's actually eligible for compensation and reimbursement. But you still continue to acquire data on its performance and you have the authority to modulate or change your regulatory decision." You would end up "with much broader access and a much more rational economic model for the developer."

We asked Dr. von Eschenbach whether what he is proposing is effectively a federal Right to Try with a program of postmarket surveillance attached. Once the drug's safety is established, it would be made broadly available early in the development process to a wide patient population and the company would then continue to collect data to improve it as it went. So the result would be the same—dying patients who currently can't get into trials could now go to their doctors and get the investigational drugs—but with the added benefit that their progress would be monitored and reported to FDA. "That's a fair interpretation," he says (though he underscored his belief that the reforms should be made at the federal level).

With the right incentives in place, says Garabedian, smart drug companies would embrace large-scale early access programs. Those who did would benefit over those who did not in a number of important ways.

First, they would get an edge on the competition. Garabedian says that expanded access would give innovative companies a chance to be the first to get their drugs into the hands of treating physicians. "These are still the ultimate customer who prescribes the drug and it allows the primary customer to get hands-on experience with a drug." He says most treating physicians are not involved in clinical trials, or have only a few patients who qualify. "In a competitive scenario, especially with products that are not significantly differentiated, the product that physicians have the most experience [with] and knowledge [of] from their hands-on application of the drug will likely have a huge advantage over [a product from] a company that doesn't widely employ an early access program."

Second, Garabedian says, "early access programs can act as a 'beta test' for what would typically happen in a commercial launch setting." Once a product is unleashed in the marketplace, he explains, there is always a significant amount of learning by the company in how the customers interact with the product. "Physicians and patients and caregivers will engage the company with various questions, highlight issues or concerns, and provide general commentary on their direct experience with the product."

Software companies do this every day. They get their product out to a sampling of the intended audience and use the feedback from these early adopters to improve the product and their marketing strategy. By getting new drugs out to medical early adopters through a broad expanded access program, a company can get that kind of feedback and can use these early experiences to improve the product and adjust its marketing strategy.

"This 'beta test' would allow the official launch to have a more successful communications and customer engagement strategy," Garabedian says. "Furthermore, this early feedback could have a direct impact on the negotiation of the package insert and label content with regulators."

Third, Garabedian says, early access would be an opportunity for companies to build goodwill—and thus brand loyalty—in the patient community. "The goodwill that an early access program would generate among the health-care provider community and patient community could be significant," he says. Patients and the doctors who treat them will never forget that a particular company fought to get them life-saving drugs in time. This would be especially valuable and attractive to companies that have multiple products in a specific disease area, and "enable a loyalty and commitment to the company for the long term."

Fourth, Garabedian says, the FDA would benefit. The information generated from wider use of expanded access programs would "make their jobs easier as it enables more information to consider a drug's approval." Regulators "will get more comprehensive data sooner and more rapid assessments of how any drug would fare to treat a given disease" that would allow the FDA to approve drugs faster.

With the right economic incentives, he says, "it seems early access programs should be a win-win for industry and regulators alike."

So if companies would benefit, patients would benefit, and even regulators would benefit, why hasn't the FDA taken these and other steps to encourage broader access to compassionate use?

Because, Dr. von Eschenbach says, the FDA has "a very risk-averse culture." He says, "The mind-set in the FDA is 'My job is first and foremost to protect the public and not let anything bad happen to them—and then, oh, by the way I'm also supposed to promote health.' Well, the truth of the matter is the reverse is really what the charge is. It's to promote and protect the public health. The first reason for the FDA to be there is to promote. And that means—promote means more rapid efficient access to lifesaving drugs and devices."

Unfortunately, his old colleague Dr. Janet Woodcock, the director of the FDA's Center for Drug Evaluation and Research, disagrees. Asked what the FDA is doing to speed drug development, Dr. Woodcock says, "It's not about speed."

But if you are dying and waiting for a drug, it *is* about speed.

"I don't agree, okay?" she says. "I'm a doctor. If I were dying I'd want—it's about quality. Okay? If I was going to try something I'd want to know it had a chance of helping me, right? There are tons of quacks out there."

She points out that most emerging drugs fail. "Eight out of ten times they probably wouldn't help because they'd be either too toxic or it wouldn't work," she says.

This is not entirely accurate. While only about 20 percent of drugs that make it out of phase I and into phase II trials are eventually approved, according to the FDA about 60 percent of drugs in phase III trials do eventually succeed. For a terminally ill patient with 100 percent chance of dying, access to a drug with a 20 to 60 percent chance of success is a big improvement. Most dying patients would gladly take a 10 percent, or a 5 percent, or even a 1 percent chance—anything above zero.

Moreover, doctors, patients, and patients' advocates are not stupid. They are not choosing drugs by throwing darts at a wall. Patients meticulously research the various treatments that are in clinical development. Doctors carefully study the results of clinical trials. They know which drugs are promising and which ones are not.

Frank Burroughs of the Abigail Alliance points out that "every drug for cancer and other serious life-threatening illnesses that we pushed for earlier access to, earlier approval of, every drug is now approved by the FDA. There's not one drug we've pushed for earlier approval of that would not be able to make it through the clinical trial process.

"I think you call that batting a thousand," he says.

Dying patients are not looking for a 100 percent guarantee the drug is effective. They are looking for hope. They are looking for a fighting chance.

Unfortunately, getting them that chance requires pressure—and sometimes it requires harnessing the power of shame. Former secretary of defense Donald Rumsfeld—the former head of G. D. Searle and chairman of Gilead Sciences—says shame is a powerful motivator. "People don't succeed in government by being anything other than risk averse. But risk-aversion tends not to include the shame factor," he says. "Shame is a killer. People don't like to be shamed. They don't like to look like jackasses even though their conduct results in jackass outcomes."

Today, social media have empowered patients to fight for themselves and draw attention to "jackass outcomes"—like the ones experienced by Mikaela Knapp, Kianna Karnes, Nick Auden, Andrea Sloan, Diego Morris, Austin McNary, and countless other Americans fighting to save their lives.

Moreover, social media are disrupting and democratizing the drug development and approval process. It used to be that drug development was a closed ecosystem, in which drug companies and the FDA had a monopoly on information. Parents in clinical trials didn't know each other, they could not compare stories of how they or their children were responding, and so they had no idea how a clinical trial was progressing.

Today, thanks to social media, if a trial is working, the word spreads at the speed of Facebook. Indeed, patients sometimes know that a drug is working before the drug companies do. Chris Garabedian says the first time he had an inkling that Sarepta's drug eteplirsen was working was when Jenn McNary came up to him at the Duchenne conference and told him her son was getting better and demanded the drug for her other son. She was online sharing that information with other Duchenne moms, who were telling similar stories. The data later confirmed what the moms already knew thanks to the power of social media.

When patients and parents know a drug is working, they are not going to sit back and wait for years for the FDA to satisfy itself with near–100 percent certitude about the efficacy of a drug. Patients are demanding action. They are demanding speed. They are demanding access. They are demanding the Right to Try.

In Europe, Ronald Brus has found a way to meet this demand, by creating an online clearinghouse that provides physicians and patients who are excluded from clinical trials access to drugs in development.

Brus was the CEO of Crucell, a Netherlands-based biotech company that produced revolutionary vaccines, when his father came down with inoperable lung cancer. He says, "Being at the heart of the industry I felt that I could fix that, right?" So he called several people in the United States and asked whether they had any new, cutting-edge drugs for lung cancer. They said yes, but he found it was impossible to get those innovative treatments to his father. Here he was, the CEO of a major biotech company—a leader in his industry, with twenty-five years in drug development—and even *he* could not get access to the experimental drugs he needed to save his father. Before his father died, he promised him he would change that.

"Like my dad, there's about over a million people a year that basically hear from the doctors that there's no treatment option left. And what they basically mean is that in their toolbox that's approved there's nothing left," he says. "But if you assume that the next iPhone is better than the iPhone that you currently have . . . you know that there is something in the pipeline that might be much better."

He sold his company, Crucell, to Johnson & Johnson for about $3 billion and together with other European biotech entrepreneurs started a new company called myTomorrows. Brus describes myTomrrows as an iTunes for investigational drugs and treatments. His company builds bridges among patients, doctors, and drug developers. Doctors and patients can go to his site and find out what drugs are in development for a particular disease, how many patients are using them, and how they rate them. Then myTomorrows helps facilitate requests for permission from governments in Europe for early access for physicians and pharmacists.

Brus is creating an economic model through which patients can benefit, and drug manufacturers can profit, from early access. "We are active in every country in Europe already," he says. Now he wants to bring his model to America—and he thinks that he will eventually be able to do so because of the pressure from the Right to Try movement.

"Because of Right to Try there's pressure on the system and the FDA needs to bend," he says. "It's like what Uber did to the cab world is put pressure on the system and say, 'Hey guys, the system was intended to protect patients but it became a system that just protects the establishment and is harmful to patients.'"

The FDA is going to have to deal with the growing demand for investigational treatments. It is going to have to accept that the information age is disrupting the model of drug development to which it and the drug companies have grown accustomed. It is going to have to change its model or face a grassroots revolution that will change the model for it.

"We have to deal with it," says Dr. Woodcock. "But people always say stuff like this but you have to realize that the drug development process is basically a scientific evaluation process, that's what it is. It's not a vote.

"Everyone in the world who talked to each other four hundred years ago believed the world was flat; it didn't mean it was flat," she says. "So science is different. The scientific process is not changing."

The FDA right now is in resistance mode. It sees those seeking earlier access and faster approval as "flat-earthers" and believes its job is to defend the scientific process against the onslaught. It sees patients, parents, and advocates as a challenge to be managed. It meets with them regularly and has them "testify" before its committees. But while it "listens" to patients, too often it does not hear—and does not act.

That is going to have to change.

The truth is that today the FDA pays lip service to compassionate use but does not really support it. When asked if it would be a good thing if hundreds of thousands of people were receiving investigational medicines on a compassionate basis, Dr. Woodcock sighs and says: "Well, it would be another burden on the health-care system."

"Another burden."

That is how FDA sees dying patients seeking compassionate access to drugs?

These patients are not a "burden." They are human beings. They are also American citizens. The FDA works for them. It is the FDA's job to help patients get access to drugs that could potentially save their lives.

Does Dr. Woodcock believe dying patients have the Right to Try?

"As I said, eight out of ten times [the drugs] probably wouldn't help because they'd be either too toxic or [they] wouldn't work. However, for those individuals who wanted to try something, definitely. We shouldn't look people in the face and say, 'Okay, you're dying and we have nothing to offer you' if there's something they could try.

"I believe that it's only fair that if you have a fatal disorder you should be able to try. We, the federal government, shouldn't stand between people who are dying and treatments they think could help them. That's what I believe," she says.

The FDA claims that it doesn't stand in the way of dying Americans' getting access. We have seen how, in a myriad of ways, it does. But "not standing in the way" is not good enough.

The bigger problem is that the FDA won't *fight* to get them access. If their own government won't fight for them, we will.

## 8.

# Would You Use a
# Fifteen-Year-Old Cell Phone?

*How to Get American Medicine Back on Top*

———

Do you remember what your cell phone looked like fifteen years ago? It was a big hunk of plastic with a large stub antenna, a black-and-white display, no camera, no video, no keyboard, no email, no text messaging, no Internet connection, no GPS, no apps, no music, and almost no memory.

If you showed it to your kids today, they would laugh and ask, "Did people really use those?"

Well, if you wouldn't use fifteen-year-old cell phone technology to make a call today, why should you be forced to depend on fifteen-year-old medical technology to save your life?

Because that is exactly what you are getting when you put the latest FDA-approved drugs into your body.

In an age when the speed of technological innovation is accelerating in almost every aspect of our lives, the time it takes to bring a new drug from the laboratory to the pharmacy shelf has nearly doubled over the last five decades. It now takes, on average, nearly fifteen years to bring a new drug to market.

This is not the fault of scientists. As we have seen, they are pioneering incredible cures and treatments for diseases from ALS to muscular dystrophy that were once unimaginable. No, the problem lies not with the innovators but with the regulators.

Today, instead of speeding medical innovation, the government is routinely slowing it down—demanding more data, more tests, and more procedures on more subjects before it will approve a drug. Clinical trials are getting longer, larger, and more complex. As a result, the cost of developing new drugs is skyrocketing, while the time it takes to get these drugs to dying patients is slowing. Even FDA commissioner Margaret Hamburg admitted in 2010, "We are left relying on 20th century approaches for the review, approval and oversight of the treatments and cures of the 21st century."[1]

What do you think your iPhone would look like if it had to go through the same regulatory process as medical treatments? Answer: you would not have an iPhone.

Today, doctors and scientists routinely come up with novel ways to treat diseases only to run into delays at the FDA.

HERE IS WHAT THE Obama administration says. In September 2012 the President's Council of Advisors on Science and Technology (PCAST) issued its "Report to the President on Propelling Innovation in Drug Discovery, Development and Evaluation." The report found:

> Evidence indicates that the time and cost for conducting clinical trials of new drug candidates is rising. Over the past 50 years, the time from drug discovery to drug approval has nearly doubled from 8 years in the 1960s to roughly 14 or more years now. More recently, some experts conclude that the time required for drug development (from patent filing to commercialization) has increased from an average of 9.7 years for drugs launched during the 1990s to an average of 13.9 years for drugs launched since 2000.
>
> Factors include the increasing complexity of clinical trial

protocols, including the procedures to be applied, the growing difficulty of recruiting and retaining patients that meet the criteria for clinical trials, the administrative burdens of setting up clinical trials, and increasing regulatory requirements for clinical trials in particular areas.[2]

The report also notes that these anti-innovation policies disproportionately affect small companies:

While the factors above are important to all innovators, they may be especially important to small biotechnology companies. When the FDA determines that the available evidence is inadequate to support approval and that additional studies are required, a large pharmaceutical firm with many products in its pipeline can accommodate the delay more readily than a small biotech firm. Small firms often have only a single drug under development. Because such companies have no commercial sources of revenue to support their high "burn rate," a two-year delay in drug approval can be a death knell.

The FDA denies that it is to blame.

"My analysis which I have pursued over many years is that the FDA is really not at the heart of this problem," says Dr. Janet Woodcock, the FDA's director of drug evaluation. The FDA, she insists, is approving new drugs and treatments at a record pace.

Writing in the newspaper *The Hill* in April 2015, Dr. Woodcock and Dr. Karen Midthun, director of the FDA Center for Biologics Evaluation and Research, claimed that the FDA had achieved "drastic reductions in the time it takes the agency to review new drugs." They claimed that the "FDA consistently reviews new drugs faster than all other advanced regulatory authorities around the world, including the European Medicines Agency."[3]

As evidence of the FDA's supposed speed, Drs. Woodcock and

Midthun point to an FDA report, "Novel New Drugs 2014 Summary," which claims that the agency "approved a majority of the novel new drugs of 2014 (32 of 41, 78%) on the 'first cycle' of review, meaning without requests for additional information that would delay approval and lead to another cycle of review."[4] In each case, the FDA claims, the drugs were "approved" in a matter of months.

This is deeply misleading. To understand why, imagine for a moment that you need to apply for a mortgage and there is only one bank in the entire world that can give it to you. So you go to the bank and tell it you want to apply for a loan. It says it needs you to go back and collect all your financial data. So you collect all the information it wants, come back, and give it to the bank. A few months later, it comes back and says: we need more data. So you go back, collect the data it wants, and give it to the bank. Then a few months later, it says: we need even more data. You give it to the bank. Then imagine the process repeats itself—over, and over, and over—until almost a decade has gone by. (There are no other banks you can go to, so you have no choice but to deal with this one bank.)

Then one day the bank finally says: Okay, we have all the information we need, you can file your loan application. So you file the application, and a few months later, the bank approves it.

And the bank says: See how fast we are! We approved your loan in just a few months!

You say: Are you kidding me? We started this process nine years ago!

That is what the FDA is doing when it comes to drug approvals.

A drug sponsor comes to the FDA and says: We have a new drug and we want to move from the lab into human trials. The FDA asks for data from laboratory testing and, if it is promising, it allows the sponsor to begin to file what is called an Investigational New Drug (IND) application and start the clinical trials. Then, as the trials go along, the FDA continues to demand more and more data each step of the way. And the drug sponsor keeps producing it—waiting for the invitation from the FDA to file the NDA. This process takes many years—sometimes a decade or more.

Then, one day, the FDA finally says: Okay, we have all the data we need, you can file a new drug application. The sponsor files the application and a few months later, the FDA approves it.

And the FDA says: See how fast we are! We approved the drug in just a few months!

In fact, the process took years.

Here is a real-life example of how misleading the FDA's statistics are. Remember the story in chapter 1 about Jenn McNary's fight to get the FDA to approve eteplirsen, the Duchenne muscular dystrophy drug her son, Austin, desperately needs? The FDA kept playing "Lucy with the football" with the drug company, Sarepta Therapeutics. For three years, the company kept providing the agency with data showing the drug was safe and effective. And for three years, the FDA kept promising Sarepta it could apply for an NDA—only to pull back the invitation and demand more data. As of April 2015, Sarepta was still waiting for the green light to submit its new drug application to the FDA.

That means, by the FDA's standards, the approval clock for eteplirsen *hadn't even started yet*.

Does anyone think the clock has not started for Jenn McNary? Her son Austin has been waiting *for years* to get access to the drug. For him, the clock has been ticking and ticking and ticking, while his condition has been declining and declining and declining.

Eteplirsen is not unique. Indeed, many of the FDA's most celebrated success stories of drugs it says were "approved" in a few months' time have in fact taken years.

Here are seven examples of drugs the FDA claims it approved in 2014 under "accelerated approval." In each case, the FDA claims it approved the drugs a matter of months. In each case, we went back into the FDA records and calculated the *actual* time it took to approve the drug from the filing of an IND application to final approval:

- **OPDIVO**—a drug to treat patients with unresectable (cannot be removed by surgery) or metastatic (widely spread) melanoma who no longer respond to other drugs.

  *FDA claimed approval time: 4 months, 22 days*

  *Actual approval time: 8 years, 5 months, 23 days*

- **LYNPARZA**—a drug to treat advanced ovarian cancer.

  *FDA claimed approval time: 10 months, 16 days*

  *Actual approval time: 8 years, 3 months, 27 days*

- **BLINCYTO**—a drug to treat patients with Philadelphia chromosome-negative precursor B-cell acute lymphoblastic leukemia (B-cell ALL).

  *FDA claimed approval time: 2 months, 14 days*

  *Actual approval time: 8 years, 3 months, 15 days*

- **KEYTRUDA**—a drug for treatment of patients with advanced or unresectable melanoma who are no longer responding to other drugs.

  *FDA claimed approval time: 9 months, 13 days*

  *Actual approval time: 4 years, 8 months, 25 days*

- **ZYDELIG**—a drug to treat patients with three types of blood cancers.

  *FDA claimed approval time: 10 months, 12 days*

  *Actual approval time: 5 years, 6 months, 22 days*

- **BELEODAQ**—a drug to treat patients with peripheral T-cell lymphoma (PTCL).

  *FDA claimed approval time: 6 months, 24 days*

  *Actual approval time: 9 years, 7 months, 18 days*

- **ZYKADIA**—a drug to treat patients with a certain type of late-stage (metastatic) non-small-cell lung cancer (NSCLC).

  *FDA claimed approval time: 4 months, 5 days*

  *Actual approval time: 3 years 6 months, 21 days*

In other words, the FDA's claims are grossly inaccurate.

And all these are cancer drugs, which are among the fastest drugs to be approved. The Neurological Division—the division reviewing Sarepta's Duchenne drugs—has not approved a single drug under accelerated approval since 2004, more than a decade.

So what can be done to speed the drug development and approval process? Here are a few ideas.

ONE SIMPLE REFORM WOULD be to make it easier, not harder, for drug companies to get follow-on drugs approved.

In theory, once Sarepta gets FDA approval for its first exon-skipping drug, eteplirsen, that should logically pave the way for the speedy approval of Sarepta's follow-on Duchenne drugs—all of which are built around the same core technology.

All Sarepta's Duchenne drugs use the same chemical backbone, which acts as the delivery vehicle that sends genetic information to the cell. In eteplirsen, scientists attach genetic information that instructs the cell to skip exon 51—which affects about 13 percent of Duchenne sufferers. But scientists can just as easily attach different genetic information to the same chemical backbone, instructing the cell to skip other missing exons.

So once the first drug using this chemical backbone is approved, logic dictates that the follow-on drugs based on the same chemical backbone should speed through FDA approval, right? If it works on exon-51, the exon Max and Austin McNary are missing, it should work on exon-53, the exon Jordan McLinn is missing.

In practice, that is not how FDA approval works. Rather than making it easier to approve follow-on therapies, the agency often makes it harder and harder for each subsequent drug to get to market.

And those delays have a terrible human price.

This is precisely what happened when the FDA considered new drugs targeting MPS diseases (mucopolysaccharidoses)—a cluster of terrible genetic disorders that cripple, and often kill, children. Children with MPS diseases are born without the ability to produce enzymes that break down certain complex molecules in the body. These molecules then accumulate in cells and tissues in places like the heart, brain, liver, joints, respiratory system, and central nervous system—disfiguring, debilitating, and eventually killing the children. The diseases—including Gaucher, Hunter, and Pompe—are extremely rare, each with only a few thousand victims.

Writing in *National Affairs*, Dr. Scott Gottlieb, a former FDA deputy commissioner and a scholar at the American Enterprise Institute, explains that in the early 1990s, the first treatments for MPS diseases began to emerge as drugs were developed that could function as replacements for the missing enzymes.[5]

The first drug, Ceredase, was designed to treat an MPS disorder called Gaucher disease, which kills most affected children before the age of five.

"Ceredase was approved by the FDA in 1991 on the basis of a single, six-month study of 12 patients," Dr. Gottlieb says. "When regulators saw that the [abnormally enlarged] livers and spleens of these patients were shrinking, the FDA took it as evidence that the replacement enzyme was having its intended clinical benefit. If the FDA had required statistically significant evidence that the drug enabled patients to function better or live longer, rather than settling for proof that it addressed the physical markers of the disease, the trial could have taken several years.

"But given the severity of the disease, as well as the absence of alternative treatments, the agency opted to approve Ceredase once the drug's safety was clearly established."

It was a good-news story. The FDA acted with speed to save dying children suffering from a rare, debilitating, and deadly illness with no other available treatment or cure.

It was an example of government working as it should.

Fast-forward a decade. Encouraged by both the success and the rapid approval of Ceredase, scientists and manufacturers have developed similar treatments for other MPS diseases. They reasonably expected that each subsequent approval would be easier and faster. After all, when the FDA approved Ceredase for Gaucher disease, it did not know whether or not restoring the missing enzyme was going to have a therapeutic effect. But now, after years of treatment, doctors were certain that if you give the enzyme to MPS patients, and the enzyme stays in the blood, the patients are going to experience a therapeutic effect, slowing or even stopping the advance of the disease.

So most people in the MPS community expected that approving the next round of enzyme-replacement drugs would be easier, not harder.

They were wrong.

Instead of speeding approval as follow-on drugs were developed, the FDA suddenly put on the brakes—holding up approvals while requiring larger, more complex, and more rigorous clinical trials.

In the early 2000s, Elaprase, a drug for another MPS condition called Hunter's syndrome, was discovered. But instead of requiring a six-month twelve-patient trial, as it had for Ceredase, this time the FDA required a yearlong trial that involved ninety-six patients with Hunter's disease—which, Dr. Gottlieb says, amounted to "some 20 percent of all Americans afflicted with the disease."

It was an exceptionally high number.

But the story gets worse. Not only did the FDA require an unreasonably large trial, but "for the first time in such a study of enzyme-replacement therapy, the FDA also insisted that patients be randomly assigned to receive either the experimental drug or an inert placebo," Dr. Gottlieb says.

That meant many families were traveling hundreds of miles in the hope that the drug would save their children from a debilitating disease—but were getting nothing more than sugar water.

This was not only cruel, Dr. Gottlieb says; it was scientifically unnecessary.

"The course of Hunter syndrome is well documented, and follows a very regular pattern in most afflicted children; the results for patients who got the experimental therapy could easily have been compared against readily available historical databases that track the normal course of the disease. It is hard to see why a placebo was necessary in such circumstances, especially when the requirement for a placebo group meant that some of the kids involved wasted a full year of the most able portion of their short lives effectively going untreated."

A decade earlier, the FDA had approved Ceredase as soon as it saw that the enlarged livers and spleens of the patients were shrinking, which it accepted as evidence that the replacement enzyme was working.

In the case of Elaprase, it had this same evidence that the drug was working eighteen weeks into the trial. According to *Science Daily*, "Liver and spleen size decreased by more than 20 percent after 18 weeks of treatment in both groups that received Elaprase, whereas liver size remained unchanged and spleen size increased in the placebo group."[6]

But instead of using that data to quickly approve the drug, the FDA insisted on letting the trial go on for a year, so it could wait to see whether the patients on the drug walked farther than patients on the placebo.

They did. When the FDA finally approved Elaprase in July 2006, the agency boasted in its news release that "patients who received Elaprase infusions experienced on average a 38-yard greater increase in the distance walked in six minutes compared to the patients on placebo."[7]

What it failed to mention was that the kids on the placebo were crippled. After a year, many couldn't walk and their breathing had declined. Even if they were eventually moved onto the drug, they would never regain all the function they had lost that year.

These were kids!

The FDA could have enrolled one hundred kids in an open-label study, given everyone the drug, and compared the results with historical databases for Hunter's disease. Instead it knowingly allowed a group of children to lose their ability to walk and breathe.

None of this was to establish the safety of the drug. It was all done, Dr. Gottlieb says, "in an effort to satisfy an increasingly unreasonable hunger for statistical certainty on the part of the FDA.

"The story of the Elaprase trial is important not because it stands out as an exception," Dr. Gottlieb continues, "but rather because it is increasingly characteristic of the FDA's drug-review culture. That culture is the product of a poorly understood, but now well-established, attitude within the agency: an excessive desire for certainty . . . [that] is impeding the availability of safe, effective drugs that could today be helping real patients."

Today, Dr. Gottlieb says, "there are currently no new treatments in clinical development for Hunter syndrome." Why? He says, "Potential new drug developers have looked at the conditions the FDA attached to the Elaprase trial and similar development procedures, and they have determined that any future studies would take too long and cost too much. Even drug makers looking at developing 'biosimilar' copies of existing drugs have so far reasoned that the process would be infeasible."

Even the original MPS drug—Ceredase—has not escaped the FDA's ever-increasing demands for statistical certainty. In 2010, when the FDA reviewed an upgraded version of the drug, Dr. Gottlieb says, "the agency required the drug to be tested in ninety-nine patients. It also wanted the drug (named VPRIV) to be tested in some patients who had not received any prior treatment for their disease. Given the availability of Ceredase, finding these 'treatment naïve' patients was no easy feat: Most people with the disease were already being treated. To find enough patients who had never been treated for the disorder required an enormous, and expensive, multiyear search that has delayed access to the medicine."

Based on this experience, anyone who thinks that once the FDA approves eteplirsen—Sarepta's drug for Duchenne patients missing exon 51—the agency is going to speed the approval of Sarepta's follow-on exons is likely in for a rude awakening.

Unfortunately, this trend is not limited to MPS drugs. The FDA is demanding more and more data, and requiring greater and greater statistical certainty, before it will approve a drug.

As a result, trials are getting larger, longer, and more complex.

According to Kenneth Getz of the Tufts Center for the Study of Drug Development, in 2012 a typical phase III trial saw an average of 170 procedures performed on each study volunteer over 230 days. Ten years earlier, the same trial required just 106 procedures over the course of 187 days.[8] That is a more than 60 percent increase in the number of procedures and a 23 percent increase in trial duration.

"Without exception we've seen a dramatic increase in the scope and demands of the study," Getz recently explained at a conference on reforming clinical trials. "The total number of end points has nearly doubled. . . . Total number of eligibility criteria has nearly doubled. . . . If you just look at the volume of data that we're collecting for a typical phase III trial today, we're approaching a million data points. . . . With every one of those data points that has to be monitored and source data verified."

Why are trials taking longer and getting more complex? Drug manufacturers fear that "failure to [follow FDA protocols] could potentially delay regulatory submission, product launch and product adoption," Getz says. The result is "higher development costs, longer study durations, and more protocol deviations and amendments."[9]

Again, almost none of this is done in the name of safety. It is in the name of guaranteeing efficacy. "What the FDA is doing is reflecting societal values," says Dr. Janet Woodcock, director of the FDA Center for Drug Evaluation and Research, in an interview.

Dr. Woodcock points out that eight out of ten drugs fail and asks what people would say if the agency had let those drugs through. Imagine, she says, "if people who build bridges . . . or skyscrapers, if they built them and eight out of ten times they fell down. That would not be good."

But the difference is that a normal person walking across a bridge expects it to work 100 percent of the time. A patient dying of ALS or cancer or some other terminal illness is not asking the FDA for a 100 percent guarantee.

She's asking for a *chance*.

"We get that," Dr. Woodcock says.

But really the FDA doesn't.

When someone has a terminal illness and has no other options, he will gladly take a drug with a 50 percent chance of 20 percent effectiveness, over the 100 percent chance that he will die without the drug.

But Dr. Woodcock protests, "If you want a 50 percent certainty that means half the drugs on the market wouldn't work. Insurance companies would be paying for them, Medicare would be paying for them, they wouldn't work."

This is what the FDA does not seem to get: dying Americans are willing to take that risk.

It can't seem to distinguish between cough medicine and a treatment for a terminal illness. When it comes to cough medicine, the FDA can take all the time in the world. No one is going to die. But when it comes to people with terminal illnesses, the FDA's often irrational quest for certainty is deadly.

. . . .

ANOTHER REFORM THAT IS needed is to put an end to the situation in which Americans like Diego Morris have to go to Europe to get a safe and effective drug that is not available here in America—by making drug approvals reciprocal, so that drugs approved in Europe are automatically available here.

It is not just cancer patients who face this dilemma.

Idiopathic pulmonary fibrosis (IPF) is a fatal lung disease with no known cure. According to the National Heart, Lung, and Blood Institute, the "tissue deep in your lungs becomes thick and stiff, or scarred, over time. . . . As the lung tissue thickens, your lungs can't properly move oxygen into your bloodstream. As a result, your brain and other organs don't get the oxygen they need."[10]

"This disease is deadlier than 60 to 70 percent of malignancies," says Dr. Daniel M. Rose, chief executive of the Pulmonary Fibrosis Foundation.[11]

Most people live only three to five years after diagnosis.

"They suffocate from their lungs filling up with Jell-O," Dr. Paul W. Noble, an IPF expert at Duke University, told an FDA advisory committee.[12]

There were no effective treatments for IPF until a drug company named InterMune developed a breakthrough therapy called pirfenidone (Esbriet) that reduces the scarring in the lungs and thus extends life. It was approved by the FDA in October 2014. The FDA hailed the approval in a press release, declaring the decision as evidence that "[w]e continue to help advance medication therapies by approving products that treat conditions that impact public health."[13]

In fact, it is evidence of the opposite.

In March 2010 four years and seven months earlier, an FDA advisory panel had recommended approval of pirfenidone, but the FDA rejected the drug.[14]

There were three clinical trials done examining its safety and effectiveness—two in the United States and one in Japan. One of the US trials showed the drug worked by a statistically significant margin, as did the Japanese trial. The second US trial just barely missed statistical significance, but the FDA advisory panel realized it was because of a flaw in the trial. Weighing the evidence of effectiveness, the safety data, and the unmet medical need, the panel voted overwhelmingly, 9 to 3, to recommend the drug for approval.

But the FDA rejected the drug. The agency said it needed two trials showing effectiveness. It had two trials, but it would not accept the Japanese trial—because all the patient-level case reports were in Japanese. So even though the drug targeted a huge unmet medical need, even though there were two studies confirming its effectiveness, and even though its own advisory committee said it believed the data, the FDA refused to make the drug available—withholding an effective treatment that was desperately needed by approximately 100,000 patients with IPF. It demanded that the company conduct yet another trial.

There was no doubt about the general safety of pirfenidone. The FDA wasn't protecting anyone. Quite the opposite: its delays were consigning many desperate patients to certain death.

On February 28, 2011, after looking at exactly the same data, the European Medicines Agency (EMA) approved the drug for use in all twenty-eight EU member states.[15] The following year, on October 1, 2012, Health Canada approved pirfenidone based on the same data. And it has been approved for use in Japan since October 16, 2008.[16]

After its European approval, the drug took off across the Continent. By 2012, 42 percent of all respiratory specialists in Europe were using pirfenidone as first-line treatment for newly diagnosed IPF.[17]

But the FDA did not finally approve the drug until October 15, 2014.

That means the FDA needlessly withheld the drug from dying Americans for three years and eight months after the European

Medicines Agency approved it. It withheld it from dying Americans for two years after Health Canada approved. It withheld it for four years and seven months after its own advisory committee voted overwhelmingly to approve it.

To understand the human costs of that decision, consider: About 40,000 Americans die each year of IPF. That means an estimated 183,000 Americans lost their lives while the FDA was withholding the only known treatment for this disease.

That should never have happened. And there is a simple solution to make sure it never happens again: The United States should institute a policy of regulatory reciprocity with countries that have a proven record of approving safe and effective drugs—including the European Union, Canada, Japan, and Australia.

As Dr. Tom Coburn—a physician, former US senator, and scholar at the Manhattan Institute's Project FDA—explains, "We ought to say if it's approved in the European Union, its approved here. If it's approved in Japan it's approved here. That would markedly lower costs and markedly increase availability of new drugs and new devices."

As Dan Klein and Alex Tabarrok, two economists at George Mason University, explain, "Such an arrangement would reduce delay and eliminate duplication and wasted resources. By relieving itself of having to review drugs already approved in partner countries, the FDA could review and investigate NDAs more quickly and thoroughly."[18]

Of course, the FDA does not see it that way. The agency resists the idea of reciprocity because, according to Manhattan Institute scholars Paul Howard and Yevgeniy Feyman, "if access to the large and lucrative U.S. market could be obtained by going to the EMA rather than the FDA, there might be a mass exodus of drug applications to the E.U."[19]

But that is precisely why we need reciprocity. If FDA officials know that drug companies can go to the EMA instead, they will be more reasonable and rational in their decision making.

Does anyone think that if FDA officials knew that InterMune could simply go to the EMA to get reciprocal approval of pirfenidone, the agency would have overturned its own advisory panel's recommendation and rejected it in 2010? That's unlikely. Many thousands of lives could have been saved.

Joe DiMasi and Christopher-Paul Milne of the Tufts Center for the Study of Drug Development, and Alex Tabarrok of George Mason University, shed some light on the FDA's culture in their 2014 *FDA Report Card*:

> The FDA faces asymmetrical incentives. Damage can occur when bad drugs are approved quickly or when good drugs are approved slowly. However, the cost to the FDA of these two outcomes is not the same. When bad drugs are approved quickly, the FDA is scrutinized and criticized, victims are identified, and their graves are marked. In contrast, when good drugs are approved slowly, the victims are unknown. We know that some people who died would have lived had new drugs been available sooner, but we don't know which people. As a result, premature deaths from drug lag and drug loss create less opposition than deaths from early approval, and the FDA's natural stance is one of deadly caution.[20]

Sam Kazman, general counsel of the Competitive Enterprise Institute, says that even the victims of FDA delays usually don't realize their own government's culpability. "All they know is that their doctors told them that nothing more could be done to help them. Only a fraction of these people will understand the reason for this— namely, that a useful drug was bottled up at FDA. Unlike in the first scenario, these people do not realize that they too are victims of FDA mistakes. Their suffering or death is simply viewed, by them and others, as reflecting the state of medicine rather than the status of an FDA drug application."[21]

Former FDA commissioner Alexander M. Schmidt once told Congress, "In all of FDA's history, I am unable to find a single instance where a congressional committee investigated the failure of FDA to approve a new drug. But, the times when hearings have been held to criticize our approval of new drugs have been so frequent that we aren't able to count them. . . . The message to FDA staff could not be clearer."[22]

Reciprocity would create a countervailing set of incentives to speed drug approvals. If the FDA did not improve its regulatory process, manufacturers could simply go to Europe, Canada, Australia, or Japan to get their drugs approved.

Critics say this might create a race to the bottom, with agencies lowering standards to attract applications and the application fees that come with them. But the fact is there are plenty of ways to protect against this. For example, as Paul Howard and Yevgeniy Feyman explain, "Reciprocity could be limited to our highly developed trading partners, and to well-understood drug classes or products where there is a high unmet need, like cystic fibrosis or the myriad cancers that don't respond well to available therapies."[23]

Moreover, as Dr. Henry I. Miller, the founding director of the FDA's Office of Biotechnology and a fifteen-year agency veteran, points out, "Reciprocity could be achieved, for example, simply by giving the FDA a finite period of time (say, 60 days) from the date of an EU, Japanese or Canadian approval to show cause why a product should not be approved. In the absence of such evidence from the FDA (which would carry the burden of proof), the drug would be approved automatically."[24]

Further, no regulatory agency—whether in Europe, Australia, Japan, or the United States—is going to grant approval to any drugs that have not passed phase I safety testing. So the question is not one of lowering the bar on safety. Rather it is how to get regulators to give promising drugs to patients facing terminal illnesses faster, without wasting years seeking near-perfect assurance of efficacy.

The FDA routinely drags its feet on the approval of drugs that are approved in Europe and advanced non-European countries. We saw this in 2013 and 2014, when several American college campuses experienced meningitis B outbreaks. According to the Meningitis Research Foundation, meningitis B "leads to death in 10% of all cases and to long-term aftereffects in a further 36%," including amputations, brain damage, and hearing loss. The US campus outbreaks took the lives of students at Georgetown University, Kalamazoo College, Princeton University, San Diego State University, and Drexel University, and caused a University of California–Santa Barbara lacrosse player to have his feet amputated. Yet many parents were stunned to learn that a vaccine for meningitis B called Bexsero, manufactured by Novartis, was approved in the European Union, Australia, and Canada—but was not available in the United States.

"Officials at the affected campuses were forced to appeal to the federal government for special permission to import and administer it," Dr. Miller says. They had to apply to the FDA for compassionate use of an unapproved drug. According to Dr. Miller, it took nine months after the first meningitis B case appeared for the FDA to get the vaccine to Princeton University and it was never made available to students at Kalamazoo College and Drexel University.

When she heard that the FDA was not going to give the drug to students at Kalamazoo, Alicia Stillman—whose daughter Emily died in the outbreak at Kalamazoo—finally had enough. She organized a bus to take dozens of college-age students across the border to Canada to have the vaccine administered in Windsor, Ontario.[25]

As Mrs. Stillman explained on Forbes.com: "Last February, my nineteen year old healthy daughter contracted the B strain while away at college. . . . She died within 30 hours of entering the hospital with a headache. My life has been changed forever. I have followed the 'compassionate release' of the Bexsero vaccine to those 'lucky' Princeton students—and can only hope the rest of us find it available soon. If any of the decision makers at the FDA watched their sweet daughter die such a death, and if those decision makers had to go choose a coffin and a headstone for one of their children, I have a feeling the decision would be made a little quicker."[26]

Emily Stillman died in February 2013. Yet it took the FDA almost two more years to finally approve Bexsero for use in the United States in January 2015.[27]

If there had been reciprocity between the EMA and the FDA, there would have been no need for American college students facing a deadly outbreak of meningitis B to wait for months to get the vaccine under compassionate use.

The problem is not limited to drugs. In November 2011 the FDA approved a revolutionary heart valve called the Sapien Transcatheter Heart Valve—the first artificial heart valve that can replace an aortic heart valve without open-heart surgery. The artificial valve is compressed into the end of a long, thin, tube slightly wider than a pencil. The tube is then inserted into the artery through a small cut in the leg and threaded up to the heart, where it is placed and released. For patients who could not have open-heart surgery, it was a lifesaving development. Clinical studies showed that after a year, almost 70 percent of patients who received the valve were alive, compared with 50 percent of those who received an alternative treatment.

As Dr. Andy von Eschenbach and Ralph Hall, a professor at University of Minnesota Law School, pointed out in the *Wall Street Journal*, "This would be a great story for American patients, but for one frustrating detail: The Sapien valve has been available in Europe since 2007, saving lives there but not here."

They added, "Unfortunately, this delay was not exceptional. American patients used to be the first to benefit from their country's enormous investments in basic medical research. Today, Americans wait as much as 60% longer than they did in 2005 for new lifesaving and life-enhancing medical devices—such as stents that keep arteries open and defibrillators—to reach the market, according to a recent Government Accountability Office report. During that wait, many remain sick or disabled. Some die."[28]

Reciprocity would have brought this revolutionary valve to the United States five years earlier.

Reciprocity would have allowed Diego Morris to get mifamurtide here at home, instead of having to move to London for nine months. Reciprocity would have made pirfenidone accessible to some 183,000 Americans who died while the FDA demanded more data in its quest for statistical certainty. Delay kills.

FINALLY, WE NEED TO adapt the drug development and approval process to the era of personalized medicine.

In the world of national security, we are experiencing what has become known as the "Revolution in Military Affairs," with new weapons so precise that they can take out a target in one floor of a building without damaging the other floors.

Today, in the world of science, we are experiencing a Revolution in Medical Affairs, with new treatments so precise that doctors can take out a patient's own cells, reprogram them, and then turn them into missiles that target disease cells without damaging healthy cells.

We saw how this works in the case of Emily Whitehead, the little girl in chapter 4 who was dying from leukemia—until doctors extracted her blood, separated out her T cells, genetically reprogrammed them to fight her cancer, and then infused them back into her body, curing her.

We are entering an era when new medical treatments will increasingly be like this—designed to fit each of our individual molecular biologies.

"Precision medicine is the future of medicine," says the Manhattan Institute's Peter Huber, the author of *The Cure in the Code*.[29] Yet the regulatory system is still clinging to antiquated twentieth-century approaches to the study and approval of drugs that cannot keep up with the revolutionary advances taking place in the field of medicine.

Earlier we talked about reducing the overreliance on large, randomized placebo controlled studies—because forcing terminally ill patients into a system in which they may get a placebo instead of a drug is morally unacceptable.

But there is another reason to modernize study design: personalized medicine. How, Huber asks, can such large, randomized placebo trials be used for "approving a custom-made drug that will be prescribed to only one patient, in whom its safety and efficacy will be largely determined by how the patient's molecular biology interacts with itself?" In this circumstance, "any scientific demonstration of both efficacy and safety must involve a single patient study."[30]

Even in larger disease groups, the old model often fails. Take breast cancer, for example. "There is no such thing as breast cancer," Huber says. "For a while we thought there were four variations as we began exploring the molecular structures of these cancers." Now, he says, scientists have discovered at least ten distinct variations.

This means you can't have a clinical trial for "breast cancer," Huber explains, because "if the molecular structure of the disease is different then you really aren't dealing with one disease, you're dealing with a bunch of different diseases. [If] you throw a drug indiscriminately at all breast cancer patients it's not going to perform well because you're actually throwing it at ten different diseases and it may do just fine against one of them but not the others."

Moreover, today, Huber says, we are learning more and more that "pharmacology isn't a science of one hand clapping. The patient's chemistry matters as much as the drug's." So not only are you trying to treat ten different breast cancers; you are doing so while interacting with an enormous number of unique personal chemistries that could affect the drug's performance as well.

This throws a giant wrench into the FDA's four-decades-old "crowd science" approach to drug development. Personalized medicine is "the antithesis of the FDA's long-standing, one-size-fits-all drug approval process," Huber says.[31] "It can't handle the complexity and torrents of data that now propel the advance of molecular medicine."[32]

This presents a major challenge for the regulatory classes in Washington, because the truth is the FDA can't regulate personal medicine the way it has traditionally regulated treatments.

The solution is to rely more on "adaptive" clinical trials—studies that are constantly changing and adapting to new information. In a traditional FDA trial, if a drug is helping only one in ten patients, it will be considered a failure and the drug rejected. In an adaptive trial, scientists take that information and use it to adapt the trial to focus on that subset of patients and figure out why they are responding while the others are not. Perhaps the researchers go out and find additional patients who are genetically similar to the patients who benefited and bring them into the study. Or perhaps they test new combinations of drugs to see if they are even more effective in the responding patients. As they explore multiple avenues, they continue to adapt and collect data and develop a set of statistically rigorous results.

For adaptive trials to work, the reins in Washington have to be loosened. Huber says that in many ways, the adaptive trial process is like Right to Try. The targeted drug would go through the standard FDA safety trials and "then—I guess roughly what your Right to Try laws would say—just get it into the hands of the experts and let them learn from there. And you can, as long as you keep gathering the data from more and more patients and that means both their molecular profiles and their clinical effects. You will build databases that just keep getting better and better at fitting the same drug to large groups of patients who will benefit from it."

The evidence is mounting that the antiquated model of large, one-dimensional placebo studies with yes/no verdicts no longer works in many cases. In 2014 the National Cancer Institute launched what it called the Exceptional Responders Initiative,[33] in which researchers are going back over a decade of "failed" clinical trials to see whether it was the drugs that failed or the FDA.

NCI researchers went through their database of early phase clinical trials in which fewer than 10 percent of the patients responded to the treatments being studied. They looked to see how many exceptional responders—"patients who have a unique response to treatments that are not effective for most other patients"—they could find.

The results were astounding. In the initial search, they discovered about one hundred exceptional responders in whom the drug in the "failed" FDA trial actually worked. They are now going back to conduct molecular testing on these patients to figure out why they responded when others didn't. The goal is to see whether the drugs that "failed" FDA testing could be resurrected to treat a genetic subgroup of patients who might respond.

One such exceptional responder is Ed Levitt, who was interviewed in a remarkable Manhattan Institute video.[34] In 2004 Levitt was diagnosed with metastatic lung cancer that had spread throughout his body. He was given just months to live. His nurse suggested he try a new drug called Iressa, which had recently been approved by the FDA. She thought it would make his final days less painful.

Instead, it cured his cancer. In days his tumors disappeared. "Within a matter of a month, he was back to normal," his wife Linda says.

"What is Iressa?" Ed asks. "Iressa is magic!"

Iressa worked on Ed because he had a genetic mutation that made his cells amenable to the drug. But the drug did not work in patients who lacked this genetic mutation. So a year later, in June 2005, the FDA withdrew its approval for Iressa, because it did not extend life in enough patients.

Rather than going back and looking at why Iressa worked in Ed and figuring out how to find other patients who might be similarly helped, the FDA took it off the market—allowing patients who were already receiving it to continue, but not allowing any others to get the drug regardless of their genetic makeup.

The decision puzzles and frustrates Ed.

"The FDA could be so great, but it chooses not to be," he says.

Now the National Cancer Institute is going out to try to find all the Ed Levitts of the world so we can find and resurrect all the drugs that the FDA dismissed as failures when it was really the antiquated clinical-trial protocols that failed.

In 2007 a Colorado company called Regenerative Sciences, LLC, developed a procedure called Regenexx to treat orthopedic injuries using stem cells derived from a patient's own bone marrow. The stem cells are removed, isolated, processed and grown over a period of a few weeks, and reinjected into the injured areas to promote healing. According to the company website, "These stem cell procedures utilize a patient's own stem cells or blood platelets to help heal damaged tissues, tendons, ligaments, cartilage, spinal disc, or bone."

In 2008 the FDA sent the company a letter directing it to stop performing the procedure because the patients' own cells "are considered drugs" and without an FDA license, "such products may be distributed for clinical use in humans only if the sponsor has an investigational new drug application in effect."[35]

The company rejected the FDA's claims. In a combative blog post titled "FDA: Your Body Is a Drug and We Want to Regulate It," the company vowed to fight, saying it was "engaged in a David and Goliath struggle over a basic civil right—who gets to regulate your body."[36]

In 2010 the FDA sued, and two years later the US District Court in Washington, DC, sided with the FDA.[37] Regenexx moved its treatment to a clinic in the Cayman Islands (but continues to offer other same-day stem-cell procedures not subject to the FDA lawsuit in the United States).

Huber says the decision was probably inevitable under current law, but the idea that the FDA can regulate people's own stem cells as a drug is absurd. "How the hell would you control a blinded randomized trial here? You could try the process, but what you're not trying is the chemistry because your stem cells are not the same as mine. . . . There's absolutely no guarantee that the combination of chemistry in how a stem cell therapy works in you will work the same way as it will in me."

Instead of trying to regulate stem cells as a drug, he says, the FDA should treat this as an opportunity to conduct adaptive trials to study this new technology. "The FDA [should] simply put out some general guidance saying, 'Look . . . we're not defining this as a drug but you have got to feed your data, you got to collect this much data and you've got to be willing to pool it, get the patient's consent and then the profession can at least learn the conditions under which these things work and let's find out why some patients respond and others don't.'"

The same advances in personalized medicine that are revolutionizing the development of new drugs are also revolutionizing the development of medical devices.

In 2012 doctors at the University of Michigan were struggling to save three newborn infants with a terminal form of tracheobronchomalacia (TBM), which causes the windpipe to periodically collapse and prevents normal breathing. According to an article in *MIT Technology Review*, "the three infant boys were each near death. They were all on ventilators. All had airways so tiny that the breaths they tried to exhale couldn't get out."[38]

The doctors came up with a novel solution. They used 3-D printers to make models of the boys' tiny airways and then used them to design custom stents, modeled to their specific anatomy, that could open their blocked airways. The doctors then printed out the custom stents with the 3-D printer and inserted them into the boys' tracheas and bronchi.

The custom devices worked. All three boys recovered and were able to go home. They did not even need follow-on procedures to remove the stents. Doctors designed the stents to gradually dissolve as the boys grew.

Dr. Glenn Green, an associate professor of pediatric otolaryngology at the University of Michigan's C. S. Mott Children's Hospital, where the devices were designed, says, "Before this procedure, babies with severe tracheobronchomalacia had little chance of surviving. Today, our first patient Kaiba is an active, healthy 3-year-old in preschool with a bright future. The device worked better than we could have ever imagined. We have been able to successfully replicate this procedure and have been watching patients closely to see whether the device is doing what it was intended to do. We found that this treatment continues to prove to be a promising option for children facing this life-threatening condition that has no cure."[39]

As he explained to a medical journal, we are now entering an era when medical devices can be made to fit an individual patient's anatomy on the submillimeter scale.

Personalized medical devices pose challenges for the FDA similar to those posed by personalized drugs. So far the agency has approved the use of these devices on an emergency basis. But the technology is in its infancy. How is the FDA going to regulate medical devices on a mass scale, where doctors are routinely designing and implanting custom stents and other devices, where no one is like any other? The development of personalized medical devices is going to challenge the established way of doing things.

As we have seen with the rapid rise of the Right to Try movement, patients are clamoring for better and faster development of cures that could save them. Encouraging follow-on drugs, embracing reciprocity, and supporting flexible, adaptive trials are simple steps the government could take to expand access to emerging drugs and help save lives.

# 9.

# If You Have the Right to Die,
# You Should Have the Right to Try

_____

In 2005 the George W. Bush administration went to the Supreme Court to challenge an Oregon law, the Death with Dignity Act. Such a statute, known as a Right to Die law, allows patients diagnosed with a terminal illness to request a prescription for a lethal dose of medication for the purpose of ending their own life.

In 2001 Attorney General John Ashcroft moved to suspend the licenses of doctors who prescribed lethal medications under the Oregon law, citing his powers under the federal Controlled Substances Act. A federal judge blocked Ashcroft's order—a move that was upheld by the Ninth Circuit Court of Appeals—setting up an epic showdown at the Supreme Court.

In 2005 the justices heard arguments in the case of *Gonzales v. Oregon* to determine the constitutionality of Ashcroft's order and the fate of the Death with Dignity Act. United States solicitor general Paul Clement argued on behalf of the Bush administration that the state of Oregon did not have the power to regulate the practice of medicine when that practice entails prescribing federally controlled substances. Oregon's senior assistant attorney general Robert Atkinson countered that Congress intended only to address recreational drug abuse when it passed the Controlled Substances Act and that because medical practices are regulated at the state level, Ashcroft's order was invalid and the Death with Dignity Act should be upheld.

"This is an issue of federalism, and the relationship between the sovereign states and the federal government," Atkinson told the justices. Congress passed the Controlled Substances Act against the "backdrop of 200 years of responsible regulation of the practice of medicine" by the states, he said, and added, "We think it's clear that Congress intended to respect the responsibility of the states to regulate their medical practices."

On January 17, 2006, the justices ruled 6 to 3 in favor of Oregon, upholding the law. Considering "the structure and limitations of federalism," the court observed that states have great latitude in regulating health and safety, including medical standards, which are primarily and historically a matter of local concern. To hold otherwise, the court said, would mark "a radical shift of authority from the states to the Federal Government to define general standards of medical practice in every locality."

So does the Supreme Court's decision in *Gonzales v. Oregon* clear the way for states to permit the use of non-FDA-approved medications to help dying patients save their own lives?

If states have the authority to protect patients' Right to Die, don't they also have the power to protect the Right to Try?

At the Goldwater Institute, we believe they do.

State Right to Try laws are based on the well-established legal principle that US states have inherent powers to regulate medical practice for terminal patients. Moreover, Right to Try laws safeguard a constitutionally protected liberty interest—the right of a terminal patient to try to save his life by trying safe, investigational treatments.

Federal regulations that violate our constitutional liberties can never trump state laws protecting those liberties. The US Constitution provides a floor of protection for individual rights, not a ceiling. As James Madison wrote in *Federalist* number 51, our system of federalism provides "a double security . . . to the rights of the people." The fifty states serve as shields for individual rights that the federal government fails to protect. And states can harness these tools to protect the most personal, intimate right of all—the right to try to save one's life.

A federal challenge to a Right to Try act would pit the concepts of federalism and individual rights against the expansive power of the federal government. While the federal government often prevails in federalism clashes with states, the current Supreme Court is the most pro-federalism court in decades—particularly when it comes to protecting individual rights related to medical treatments.

Essential to this appeal to federalism is the fact that the Right to Try is inseparable from the concept of liberty. The Supreme Court has acknowledged that individuals have a constitutionally protected liberty interest in refusing unwanted medical treatment.[1] A patient's autonomy interest should be the same when she chooses to seek investigational treatment to fight for her life.

Support for Right to Try laws comes from the due process clauses of the Fifth and Fourteenth Amendments as well as the Ninth and Tenth Amendments to the US Constitution. The right to medical self-preservation is so "deeply rooted in the Nation's history and tradition" and "implicit in the concept of ordered liberty" that its regulation by the FDA violates fundamental rights. In other words, the right to self-preservation is a liberty so inherent and vital that no government can place limitations on it through regulation or otherwise.

The Supreme Court has never addressed the issue of investigational medication in the context presented by Right to Try.

Some critics of Right to Try point to the 1979 case *United States v. Rutherford*, in which the Supreme Court held that the government has an interest in regulating unsafe drugs.[2] But that case involved not a promising treatment that had passed FDA safety trials, but rather an ineffective drug called laetrile that the FDA had declared "a public health menace."[3]

The FDA called laetrile a "highly toxic product that has not shown any effect on treating cancer."[4] According to the National Cancer Institute, laetrile mimics "the signs and symptoms of cyanide poisoning. These include: Nausea and vomiting; Headache; Dizziness; Blue color of the skin due to a lack of oxygen in the blood; Liver damage; Abnormally low blood pressure; Droopy upper eyelid; Trouble walking due to damaged nerves; Fever; Mental confusion; Coma; Death."[5]

The concerns for safety expressed by the Supreme Court in *United States v. Rutherford* do not apply in the case of Right to Try laws. Under Right to Try, terminally ill patients can access investigational drugs *only* if they have (1) passed an FDA-approved safety trial and (2) are still actively being developed in a clinical trial under the FDA umbrella. In other words, the law relies heavily on the FDA's expertise and diligence and does not permit access to any drugs (like laetrile) that the agency has deemed unsafe. Right to Try simply extends to all terminally ill patients the same opportunities as those lucky enough to enroll in clinical trials.

Indeed, it is the very lack of access to safe investigational treatments that is actually driving dying patients into the hands of those promoting quack cures.

For example, today—thirty-six years after the *Rutherford* decision—a clinic called Oasis of Hope is still offering laetrile treatment for desperate American cancer patients across the border in Mexico. The clinic conducts admissions at the San Diego airport. "We will pick you up at the baggage claim of your choice in a van and bring you to the hospital so there is no car to rent, no hotel expense, no food to buy, and you get a private room with two beds so a Companion can come with you," the website promises.[6]

Current FDA policy drives terminally ill patients to clinics like Oasis of Hope. Right to Try laws help dying Americans get treatments the FDA says are safe enough for clinical trials, which means desperate patients are less likely to pursue dangerous ones like laetrile. If anything, there is a public safety interest in upholding Right to Try laws.

Another case that is often incorrectly cited as evidence that Right to Try laws will be struck down is *Abigail Alliance v. von Eschenbach*.[7] This case was brought in 2006 by Frank Burroughs, the Virginia dad whose daughter Abigail died after she was unable to get access to an investigational cancer drug called Erbitux. The drug was later approved by the FDA. Frank went on to form the Abigail Alliance for Better Access to Developmental Drugs to help others like Abigail get the drugs they need before the clock runs out.

The Abigail Alliance sued the FDA, arguing that terminally ill patients with no remaining FDA-approved treatment options have a constitutionally protected due process right to seek access to investigational medications that the FDA concedes are safe and promising enough for substantial human testing.

A three-judge panel of the US Circuit Court of Appeals for the District of Columbia agreed with the Abigail Alliance and ruled that the Constitution did guarantee terminally ill patients the right to seek access to experimental drugs without government permission. After the FDA petitioned the court for a rehearing, the full circuit court reversed the decision of the three-judge panel, finding there is no fundamental right to access unapproved experimental drugs, even for the terminally ill. The Supreme Court declined to hear the Abigail Alliance's appeal, leaving the lower court ruling in place.

Case closed, say Right to Try's opponents.

When asked if patients have a "right" to try, Dr. Janet Woodcock of the FDA says, "Well, I believe that was litigated in court."

Not so fast.

First of all, since the Supreme Court has not decided the issue, the question of whether terminally ill patients have a fundamental right to seek access to investigational medicine has not yet been settled. The *Abigail Alliance* decision is not binding outside the DC Circuit. The DC Circuit, while influential, is only one of twelve regional circuits, and none of the other circuit courts are required to follow it.

Second, many legal scholars believe that the DC Circuit's decision is wrong and that later decisions will go the other way. Indeed, Judge Judith Rogers and Chief Judge Douglas Ginsburg dissented and explained very thoroughly in a twenty-nine-page opinion why their colleagues were wrong:

> In the end, it is startling that the oft-limited rights to marry, to fornicate, to have children, to control the education and upbringing of children, to perform varied sexual acts in private, and to control one's own body even if it results in one's own death or the death of a fetus have all been deemed fundamental rights covered, although not always protected, by the Due Process Clause, but the right to try to save one's life is left out in the cold despite its textual anchor in the right to life. This alone is reason the court should pause about refusing to put the FDA to its proof when it denies terminal patients with no alternative therapy the only option they have left, regardless of whether that option may be a long-shot with high risks.

Among other arguments, they explained that both the common law and the Constitution support a fundamental right to "medical self-defense."[8] Self-defense is about the most firmly settled "fundamental right" that there is. So if the government wants to infringe on that right, it must show an extremely compelling reason.

Moreover, the Supreme Court has supported the right of medical autonomy in abortion, so by that logic, it should do the same when it comes to investigational drugs. The esteemed UCLA law professor Eugene Volokh explains the principle at stake here in the *Harvard Law Review*, using examples of two women:[9]

> Alice is seven months pregnant, and the pregnancy threatens her life; doctors estimate her chance of death at 20%. Her fetus has long been viable, so Alice no longer has the Roe/Casey right to

abortion on demand. But because her life is in danger, she has a constitutional right to save her life by hiring a doctor to abort the viable fetus. She would have such a right *to a therapeutic abortion even* if the pregnancy were only posing a serious threat to her health, rather than threatening her life. . . .

Ellen is terminally ill. No proven therapies offer help. An experimental *drug* therapy seems safe, because it has passed Phase I FDA testing, yet federal law bars the therapy outside of clinical trials because it hasn't been demonstrated to be effective (and further checked for safety) through Phase II testing. . . .

It can't be that a woman has a constitutional right to protect her life using medical procedures, but only when those procedures kill a viable fetus. . . . The Supreme Court has so far recognized the medical self-defense right only in abortion cases. Yet the right can't logically be limited to situations in which the defensive procedure is abortion, and rejected when a woman needs to defend herself using experimental drugs.

Moreover, Volokh says, Americans have an even broader right to lethal self-defense. It is commonly accepted that self-defense is an exception to criminal laws against murder. "Lethal self-defense is allowed even against those who threaten your life with little or no moral fault." So, Volokh writes, "if I may kill a human or an animal to protect my life, why shouldn't I be presumptively free to protect my life using medical procedures that don't involve killing, such as . . . the use of experimental drugs?

"Medical self-defense," Volokh declares, "is a constitutional right."

We believe that this is one of several arguments that would prevail if the Right to Try is brought before the Supreme Court.

The Right to Try movement is in many ways a direct response to the DC Circuit *Abigail Alliance* majority's invitation to lawmakers to safeguard the Right to Try through the democratic process:

Although in the Alliance's view the FDA has unjustly erred on the side of safety in balancing the risks and benefits of experimental drugs, this is not to say that the FDA's balance can never be changed. The Alliance's arguments about morality, quality of life, and acceptable levels of medical risk are certainly ones that can be aired in the democratic branches, without injecting the courts into unknown questions of science and medicine. Our Nation's history and traditions have consistently demonstrated that the democratic branches are better suited to decide the proper balance between the uncertain risks and benefits of medical technology, and are entitled to deference in doing so. . . . Our holding today ensures that this debate among the Alliance, the FDA, the scientific and medical communities, and the public may continue through the democratic process.

That is exactly what the Right to Try movement has done. Supporters of the Right to Try are now using the democratic process to expand access to investigational medicines—by going to the state legislatures, to which courts have generally deferred when it comes to regulating the practice of medicine.

A complementary reform is for Congress to pass legislation explicitly protecting state Right to Try laws. In July 2015, Republican representatives Matt Salmon and Paul Gosar of Arizona and Marlin Stutzman of Indiana introduced a federal Right to Try Act, which would bar the federal government from interfering with states and parties using properly enacted Right to Try laws.[10]

The Goldwater Institute is also asking the FDA to explain to the American people how it decides who gets access to investigational medicines and who does not.

In chapter 5 we learned how an American medical missionary, Dr. Kent Brantly, contracted Ebola while caring for patients in Liberia and was given an antiviral drug called ZMapp. The FDA never publicly explained how it decided to make this drug, which had never even been tested in human beings, available for use, while denying millions of Americans access to other promising drugs that actually have passed FDA safety trials.

So in August 2014, we filed a Freedom of Information Act Request seeking information about the FDA's decision-making process on the experimental Ebola drug. The FDA denied the request, claiming that releasing the records would reveal the drugmakers' trade secrets (even though we asked for no proprietary commercial information). We appealed to the Department of Health and Human Services, which also denied our request. So in June 2015, we filed a lawsuit in the US District Court in Arizona, arguing that the FDA's arbitrary withholding of this public information violates federal law and undermines the public's right to know how the government makes decisions on life-and-death matters.

Americans deserve transparency. They should not have to beg their government for the right to save their own lives, or stand by while the government makes decisions behind a veil of secrecy that allow some to live and leave others to die.

As we go to press, the FDA has not challenged Right to Try laws. It would be unwise to do so. If it does, it will lose twice—once in the court of law, and once in the court of public opinion.

All FDA enforcement litigation must be brought by the Department of Justice, which means the decision whether to bring a lawsuit to stop Right to Try is up to the attorney general and, ultimately, the president of the United States.

Any president who goes to court to try to take away the rights of dying patients to save their own lives will pay a huge political price. In this book, we have seen up close the human tragedy that takes place when people with terminal illnesses are denied their right to try. A Supreme Court fight would draw national attention to stories like these and shine a bright spotlight on the myriad ways the federal government fails dying Americans.

The more attention these cases get, the more popular Right to Try will become. Already, Right to Try laws are passing in the states by overwhelming margins. It's not hard to see why. Almost every American has lost a friend or loved one to a terminal illness or knows someone who has—and every one of us can imagine ourselves in a similar circumstance. For most of us, the answer is simple: of course we have the right to try to save our own lives. Those fighting to stop us from doing so will emerge from that fight diminished, whatever the legal outcome.

But if the powers that be in Washington do decide to take on this losing battle, they can rest assured that Goldwater Institute is prepared to defend Right to Try in court. And our record shows that we are a formidable legal adversary.

We will stand up to defend the right of dying Americans to try to save their own lives.

If the powers that be in Washington want to take us—and the millions of Americans we represent—on, that is fine by us.

They have the right to try.

# 10.

# Where Do I Start?

*A Step-by-Step Guide to Seeking an Investigational Treatment*

————

If you're among the majority of Americans who cannot participate in a clinical trial, and you'd like to try an investigational medicine or treatment, the following information may help you.

I wish I could tell you that the process will be simple and easy, because it should be. For a patient fighting for his or her life, the process should be as quick and accessible as getting any other prescription or treatment from your doctor. I also wish I could tell you that Right to Try laws have cleared away all the institutional barriers created in Washington, DC, to patients seeking access. As we have seen in this book, many of these barriers still exist. And because Right to Try laws are brand-new, and doctors and manufacturers are still figuring out how to use the law, you may need an attorney to help you navigate the process.

## Am I eligible?
The Right to Try laws vary slightly from state to state, so you'll need to check the requirements where you live. The website righttotry.org contains an up-to-date list of Right to Try laws. If your state hasn't yet adopted a Right to Try law, you may be able to exercise your Right to Try in a different state.

Eligibility requirements generally include the following: you have a terminal diagnosis; no treatment is available, or you have exhausted the standard treatments for your condition; you aren't eligible for a clinical trial; your doctor has advised you that the use of an investigational treatment is the best medical option to extend or save your life; the investigational treatment has successfully completed basic safety testing (phase I clinical trials) and is in the development pipeline as part of the FDA's ongoing evaluation and approval process; you are willing to provide "informed consent," acknowledging the potential risks associated with the use of the drug; and the company developing the treatment is willing to make it available.

**How can my doctor and I learn more about emerging treatments that could help me?**

Patient support and advocacy groups for particular conditions often receive up-to-date information on cutting-edge research and treatments. The following is a list of groups and resources that share information on emerging treatments and clinical trials:

The Abigail Alliance for Better Access to Developmental Drugs
8881 White Orchid Place, Lorton, VA 22079
Email: frankburroughs@abigail-alliance.org
Phone: (703) 646-5306
Website: www.abigail-alliance.org

AIDSinfo
PO Box 4780
Rockville, MD 20849-6303
Email: ContactUs@aidsinfo.nih.gov
Phone: (800) 448-0440
Main website: www.aidsinfo.nih.gov

Trials website: www.aidsinfo.nih.gov/clinical-trials
Twitter: @AIDSinfo

Alzheimer's Disease and Education Referral Center (at the National
Institutes of Health's National Institute on Aging)
31 Center Drive, MSC 2292, Bethesda, MD 20892
Email: adear@nia.nih.gov
Phone: (800) 438-4380
Website: www.nia.nih.gov/alzheimers
Twitter: @Alzheimers_NIH

The Center for Information and Study on Clinical Research
Participation
56 Commercial Wharf East, Boston, MA 02110
Contact form: www.ciscrp.org/about-ciscrp/contact-us
Phone: (877) MED-HERO
Main website: www.ciscrp.org
Clinical trial database website: www.ciscrp.org/programs-events/
search-clinical-trials/search
Custom clinical trial search website: www.ciscrp.org/
programs-events/search-clinical-trials
Twitter: @CISCRP

ClinicalTrials.gov (National Library of Medicine)
8600 Rockville Pike, Bethesda, MD 20894
Email: custserv@nlm.nih.gov
Phone: (888) 346-3656
Website: www.clinicaltrials.gov

MedlinePlus (National Library of Medicine)
8600 Rockville Pike, Bethesda, MD 20894

Email: custserv@nlm.nih.gov
Main website: www.nlm.nih.gov/medlineplus
Website: www.nlm.nih.gov/medlineplus/clinicaltrials.html
Twitter: @medlineplus

National Cancer Institute
9609 Medical Center Drive, Bethesda, MD 20892-9760
Contact form: www.cancer.gov/contact/email-us
Phone: (800) 422-6237
Main website: www.cancer.gov
Website: www.cancer.gov/about-cancer/treatment/clinical
    -trials/search
Twitter: @theNCI

National Heart, Lung, and Blood Institute "Children in Clinical
    Studies"
PO Box 30105, Bethesda, MD 20824-0105
Email: ResearchAndKids@nhlbi.nih.gov
Phone: (301) 592-8573
Main website: www.nhlbi.nih.gov
Website: www.nhlbi.nih.gov/childrenandclinicalstudies/index.php
Twitter: @nih_nhlbi

National Institute on Aging "Clinical Trials and Older People"
31 Center Drive, MSC 2292
Bethesda, MD 20892
Email: niaic@nia.nih.gov
Phone: (800) 222-2225
Main website: www.nia.nih.gov
Website: www.nia.nih.gov/health/publication/clinical-trials
    -and-older-people

National Institutes of Health "Clinical Trials and You"
9000 Rockville Pike, Bethesda, MD 20892
Email: NIHinfo@od.nih.gov
Phone: (301) 496-4000
Main website: www.nih.gov
Website: www.nih.gov/health/clinicaltrials
Twitter: @NIH

ResearchMatch
Contact form: www.researchmatch.org/contact
Website: www.researchmatch.org
Twitter: @ResearchMatch

## What does my doctor need to do?

Your doctor should contact the drug manufacturer to request access to an emerging treatment.

## What does the drug manufacturer need to do?

If a company agrees to provide a treatment, it can work with your doctor to provide it to you under your doctor's supervision.

## How do I pay for treatment?

Many companies provide investigational treatments to patients at no charge or at cost. Unfortunately, most insurance companies will not pay for investigational treatments as of this writing. The following groups may be able to assist with the cost of care, including treatments and travel:

Air Charity Network
Phone: (877) 621-7177
Website: www.aircharitynetwork.org

Twitter: @AngelFlightSE
Angel Flight for Veterans
6324 Culverhouse Court, Gainesville, VA 20155
Email: info@angelflightveterans.org
Phone: (800) 550-1767
Website: www.angelflightveterans.org

Corporate Angel Network
Westchester County Airport
One Loop Road, White Plains, NY 10604-1215
Email: info@corpangelnetwork.org
Phone: (914) 328-1313
Website: www.corpangelnetwork.org

Edmond J. Safra Family Lodge at National Institutes of Health
65 Center Drive, Bethesda, MD 20892
Email: cc-famlodge@cc.nih.gov
Phone: (301) 496-6500
Website: www.clinicalcenter.nih.gov/familylodge

Mercy Medical Angels
4620 Haygood Road, Ste. 1, Virgina Beach, VA 23455
Email: info@MercyMedical.org
Phone: (757) 318-9174
Website: www.mercymedical.org
Twitter: @MercyMedical

Miracle Flights for Kids
2764 N. Green Valley Pkwy. #115, Green Valley, NV 89014-2120
Email: info@miracleflights.org
Phone: (800) FLY-1711

Website: www.miracleflights.org
Twitter: @miracleflights

National Association of Hospital Hospitality Houses
PO Box 1439, Gresham, OR 97030
Email: jdavis@hhnetwork.org
Phone: (800) 542-9730
Website: www.nahhh.org

National Patient Travel Center
4620 Haygood Rd, Ste. 1, Virginia Beach, VA 23455
Contact form: www.patienttravel.org
Phone: (800) 296-1217
Website: www.patienttravel.org

Patient Advocate Foundation
421 Butler Farm Road, Hampton, VA 23666
Email: cpr@patientadvocate.org
Phone: (800) 532-5274
Website: www.patientadvocate.org
Twitter: @PatientAdvocFou

Right to Try Foundation
Email: board@righttotryfoundation.com
Phone: (801) 400-8160
Website: www.righttotryfoundation.com
Twitter: @_RightToTry
For more information, please contact the Goldwater Institute at
info@goldwaterinstitute.org or visit www.goldwaterinstitute.org.

# Afterword

*Everyone Deserves the Right to Try: An Update on Jenn McNary, Ted Harada, and Diego Morris*

---

After three years and three months of fighting, Jenn McNary finally succeeded in getting her son Austin into a clinical trial for eteplirsen.

"The FDA finally allowed the company to expand their trials to include a few older children," she says. "I think it was specifically done because they wanted us off their backs."

But on the day Austin was to get his first infusion—the day Jenn had been fighting for, hoping for, praying for—she could not be there. She had to get on a plane and take Max to Columbus, Ohio, for his six-month lab test.

So Christine McSherry, her friend and partner in the fight to get eteplirsen approved, offered to take Austin to the hospital to get the drug for the first time.

After Jenn boarded the flight to Ohio, Christine's phone rang.

It was Chris Garabedian, the CEO of Sarepta.

"I understand Austin is getting his first infusion today," he said.

"Yeah, I'm on my way in," Christine said.

"Can you pick me up, because I really want to be there too," Chris said.

"Really?" Christine said. She was floored.

"Yeah, I just got off a red-eye from Arizona. If I can be there when the first nonambulatory boy get his dose, I'd really like to do that."

Chris had flown across the country just to be by Austin's side when he finally got the drug.

"Yep, I'll pick you up," Christine said.

She got Chris and took him to the hospital, where Austin was infused—the first new patient to receive eteplirsen since the twelve-patient study began in 2011.

Why was it so important for Garabedian to be there?

"Jenn McNary was the first mom who was convinced the drug was working," he says. "The fact that she waited more than two years from that original request to get Austin on the drug, and channeled all of her energy into advocacy for accelerated approval so that all the boys who could benefit from eteplirsen could get access, was truly heroic in my eyes."

So how is Austin doing?

"He's been on the drug for eighteen weeks," Jenn says. It usually takes about six months for the drug to have a discernible impact, but Jenn already sees signs that the drug is helping.

"He's able to take his sweatshirt off without assistance and is starting to be able to write a little bit." Austin is also playing drums in his school band. "The other night he was drumming up a storm," Jenn says.

She understands that the drug won't reverse the decline Austin experienced while fighting for access.

"It's not going to make him walk again, but it really could stabilize his progression so he doesn't get worse."

And that is what is so tragic about the delay. Austin waited 170 weeks before he could finally get on the drug. For 170 weeks he watched his brother get better while he slowly got worse.

What was the cost of that more than three-year wait?

"The skills he has lost while his brother has been on drugs have been really important life skills," Jenn says.

He lost the ability to transfer himself from chair to bed, from chair to toilet, the ability to wash his hair, the ability to dress himself, cut his own food, pick up his dog, open most doors. Skills he [was] on the verge of losing [included] feeding himself, lifting his cell phone to his ear, lifting his arms for a hug, rolling to his side in bed.

The most frustrating part of the FDA is that they already have the tools that they need to be able to approve a drug like this. So we weren't asking them to do something that was against the rules, against the law, and we weren't asking them to make an exception. They've given that guidance to allow [Sarepta] to file [for accelerated approval] and then taken it back three times.

Every time the drug company got to a place where they had the data that they thought they needed to file for approval, the FDA changed their mind and moved the goalpost again. They said, "Okay, now we want more [data], or now we want different [data], or now we want more kids enrolled, we want more end points; we want you to measure the dystrophin differently."

The FDA's delays did not affect only Austin, she says. Max and the other eleven boys in the first clinical trial have had to undergo repeated surgeries just to take biopsies of their muscle tissue to test whether the treatment was helping them produce dystrophin, the missing protein that causes Duchenne.

"The FDA was not happy with the first three muscle biopsies that were taken from the kids so they asked these twelve children to go for a fourth muscle biopsy," Jenn says. It is major surgery that has no health benefits for the boys. "They're fully under anesthesia, intubated; this is a huge surgery to take a piece of muscle, which is exactly the thing that these kids are losing."

None of this was to ensure the safety of the drug; it was all to get as close as possible to absolute certainty about the drug's efficacy before the FDA approved its release.

"We have a safe and effective drug. We have a drug company that's ready to move forward. We have laws that Congress has given them in order to allow them to approve this drug under accelerated approval and they're just refusing to do it."

Jenn thinks the FDA finally gave in and created a trial for which Austin qualified in hopes of shutting her up.

"Here's what we think happened. We think the FDA got sick of hearing from us. . . . So what they did was they said, Listen, we'll just do a 'safety' trial on these older boys. You can just prove that it's safe in them. [The plan was] getting my kid on the drug so the FDA didn't have to hear from me as much."

If that was the plan, it didn't work.

"Little did they know I wasn't going to stop," Jenn says. "We didn't even pause to get excited about it. Our kids were on the drug, and we were back to the FDA a week later and said, 'Great, when are you going to approve it, because that's what we're looking for.' They thought they were going to get rid of us when our kids were on the drug but that didn't happen."

In April 2015 Chris Garabedian resigned as CEO of Sarepta—a casualty of the company's struggles with the FDA.[1]

A few weeks later, on May 19, 2015, the FDA invited Sarepta to submit a new drug application that year—a process that was completed on June 26. The company requested "priority review," which could shorten the review period from ten months to about six.[2]

"I'm cautiously optimistic," Christine says. "I analogized it to a bad relationship yesterday—'Oh man, I've been down this road before, is it going to happen again?' But the fact that they're already taking parts of the NDA tells us that it sounds like they're pretty serious about it. . . . I'm just so nervous to get excited because I don't want the disappointment again."

If all goes well, and the drug is finally approved, it will be because an innovative CEO and a group of moms joined forces to fight for faster approval.

Yet even if the FDA does finally approve eteplirsen, the drug's roller-coaster path through the FDA approval process remains a cautionary tale.

"This is the classic story," Garabedian says. "Once a drug moves forward and it's successful, everybody forgets about the delays, the inefficiency of the process, what boys could have been helped if this were approved a year ago. Nobody ever talks about that, they only talk about 'Wow! The FDA did the right thing in the end. The FDA is letting the drug move forward. Wow!' But everybody quickly has short-term memory and doesn't remember that we were right more than two years ago when we were describing the merits of why this should be considered for accelerated approval."

He points out that even if eteplirsen is approved, the fight is not over. Eteplirsen helps just 13 percent of Duchenne patients who are missing exon 51. But the company has a suite of follow-on drugs that use exactly the same chemical backbone to treat Duchenne patients with other missing exons—boys like Jordan McLinn, the young fireman in Indiana.

Will the FDA speed approval of those follow-on drugs based on its approval of eteplirsen? Or will it put those Duchenne patients through the same delays that Jenn McNary and her family suffered, or worse?

If it does the latter, the FDA will face a patient backlash that will make the fight over eteplirsen look mild by comparison.

"Now that 13 percent of the Duchenne community may get access to the drug, imagine the other 87 percent who now feel left on the sidelines," Garabedian says. "I mean, eteplirsen advocates are going to look small and feeble compared to those who might get activated who aren't going to get access to eteplirsen."

Jenn McNary and Christine McSherry will stay in the fight until all Duchenne patients get access to the drugs they need to save their lives.

Christine is amazed by Jenn's resilience and determination. She recalls coming back from one of their many trips to Washington, DC, sitting on the plane and looking at Jenn—and thinking about all the Duchenne groups that wanted nothing to do with her.

"[Here was this] mom who got pregnant at eighteen and had two kids before she was twenty-two. Dropped out of high school. Never went to college. Yet, here is this girl. . . . She was the catalyst and initiated change and a movement far beyond [what] all those other organizations [achieved]. She really did. And it just didn't matter what her education was. It might have even been her lack of education that allowed her to get out front and do that. It was just sheer passion that she had to fight for her son."

For her part, Jenn says simply, "Everybody deserves to be involved, and not feel helpless, and not feel like they have to be quiet."

You can be sure of this: Jenn McNary won't be quiet until every boy with Duchenne gets access to the drugs he needs to save his life.

On February 25, 2013, two and a half years after first being diagnosed with ALS, Ted Harada walked into a hearing room at the Food and Drug Administration headquarters in Silver Spring, Maryland, and took his seat at the witness table.

Before him on the dais sat the leadership of the FDA—the men and women who had the power to grant or deny other dying patients access to the treatment that had saved his life.

"My name is Ted Harada," he began. "I am an ALS patient and advocate. In the eight-plus hours that this meeting will take place, five people in the United States will die from ALS, and five more will be diagnosed with their death sentences."

The doctors who saved his life, Harada told the panel, have "only been allowed to treat fifteen people in three-plus years. I don't think that treating fifteen people goes hand in hand with the concept of doing everything you can for ALS patients."

He acknowledged that the FDA approval process was the "gold

standard." But, he said, "while the FDA applies its universal gold standard, eighteen thousand people have died from ALS since the trial inception in January 2010. Nearly twelve thousand people have died from ALS since I was helped after my first surgery in March 2011.

"I had a chance. I have hope. What about everyone else?"

Ted Harada had transitioned from ALS victim to ALS advocate—from patient number 11 to a champion for patients everywhere, and not just those suffering from ALS.

But he was only getting started.

"After I testified at the FDA, I didn't see a whole lot of change," Ted says. So he used some contacts at the ALS foundation to get himself appointed to an official FDA patient advisory group. He began attending meetings at FDA headquarters, but he didn't seem to be making much progress there either. He found FDA officials defensive. They spent their time trying to convince him that the drug-approval process was just fine.

Then, one day, Ted was online looking at the Neuralstem website—he often checked CEO Richard Garr's blog for updates on how the clinical trial was doing—when he came across a blog post from Garr discussing the first Right to Try legislation that was then being considered by the Arizona legislature.

So Ted started looking into Right to Try—and the more he learned, the more sense it made.

"Right now, I don't need another treatment," Ted says. "But what happens when I do? Why should the FDA even have an opportunity to tell me no? If I have a treatment that's proven, that's helped me two different times, why should I have to even ask and give the federal government the opportunity to tell me no?"

This, he decided, would be his cause.

"I tried to exert outside pressure on the FDA from my testimony. I tried to exert internal pressure from being part of the FDA representative program."

Now, he says, he has a new strategy: "I'm going to circumvent [the FDA] through Right to Try."

Ted decided to write an op-ed for his local paper, the *Atlanta Journal-Constitution*. He shared his miraculous story in print for the first time, and declared, "I am making it my personal mission to introduce 'Right to Try' to the Georgia General Assembly as part of next year's legislative session. . . . I appreciate that the FDA is the gold standard in drug safety; however, if you or a loved one were facing mortality, would you be willing to settle for a silver standard?"

After his op-ed ran, state representative Mike Dudgeon emailed Ted and told him he would be happy to sponsor the legislation. Ted connected Dudgeon with us at the Goldwater Institute, where we shared a draft of our model legislation and some of the bills that had been passed in other states.

Soon Dudgeon introduced House Bill 34, the Georgia Right to Try Act.

Ted began lobbying for the bill, writing to legislators and meeting with the legislative staff to educate them about Right to Try. He recruited another ALS patient in the Neuralstem study, Ed Tessaro, to join him in lobbying for Right to Try in Georgia.

A retired Macy's executive, Ed was in Bangkok running a marathon seven years ago when he first noticed something was wrong. "I was running a race there and for the first time in my life, after a lifetime of running, my left leg was performing differently. I had a little flutter in it and it wasn't landing solid," he says.

When he got home to Atlanta, he went to a doctor who diagnosed spinal stenosis. "I was so happy to get that news, that it was a fixable thing, I didn't even get a second opinion," Ed says. "I just said let's go fix that."

He had spinal-fusion surgery in February 2009. It didn't work.

"Four months later I was getting worse—weaker in my legs—and then I became worried again and went to see a neurologist."

He was diagnosed with ALS. "It just knocked the crap out of me because I've been a cyclist and a runner and a mountain climber for my entire life and you think you're bulletproof at that level and all of a sudden I get this."

He and Ted had lumbar surgery a month apart. Because they responded so well, they were then among the three patients who got a second round of surgery in the upper spinal area that controls breathing.

Ed did not have the dramatic reversal of symptoms that Ted experienced—no one has yet. But he is now stable in his disease, and for an ALS patient stability is life transforming. "I can still walk a hundred yards with crutches, but I have a wheelchair," he says. But five years after his ALS diagnosis, he has retained 100 percent of his lung function thanks to the surgery. "It's breathing difficulties that eventually kill you," he says, adding, "I'm in great shape. I'm the best-conditioned guy with a fatal disease you've ever seen.

"Nobody really understands ALS," he says. "They don't understand what it feels like to be a prisoner in your own body. You know, your mind works, your eyes work, you're a hundred percent sharp but you can't move, you can't speak. I mean that is a terror of a life sentence to be a prisoner in your own body."

He has testified four times before the Georgia legislature in support of Right to Try.

Ed says he told the lawmakers, "You have to look at this as a patient rights bill. I don't want you to give me a thing, I don't want a tax dollar. I don't want anybody to do anything except allow me to take a risk to save my own life, to give me a chance at an experimental therapy or drug to save my own life.

"We like experimental. We're not afraid of the word 'experimental,'" Ed told the legislators. "It's a personal sovereignty thing. We know that something's safe but we know it's 'experimental only' and we're three years away from knowing whether or not I could buy it or ask my insurance company to buy it as a therapy. Well, I don't have three years. I'll foot the bill to do it right now."

Ted was recently invited to join the national board of the ALS Association and now flies to Washington several times a year to lobby Congress. He has spoken at bioethics symposia and high school science classes, and he has helped patients in Indiana and Kansas get Right to Try introduced in their states.

"Ted is like an unstoppable force now," says Neuralstem CEO Richard Garr, who follows Ted's medical and political progress with pride.

The admiration is mutual. "He's a brave, good man. He cares," Ted says of Garr. Ted says that when he recently completed his third ALS walk, Garr flew to Georgia just to join him. "He donated to my walk team. How many people do that? How many people do that?"

He plans to keep doing the ALS walk every year. "It's two and a half miles and it wears me out," he says. "It takes a few days for my legs to recover but I can do it. And as long as I can do it, I'm going to keep doing it."

He says his wife told him this year that maybe he should skip the walk.

"And I'm like, 'Why? I can still walk.' She goes, 'I know, but do you see yourself the next few days afterward?' But I said as long as I can it's a symbol that I can still do this. And I think sometimes it provides a little hope for other people too. In the ALS community hope has been a nonexistent commodity. It doesn't exist. So if this story, and me being able to do the walk, provides just an inkling of hope, then I'll deal with [the] few days that it takes to recuperate to provide that kind of hope."

At this writing, Ted's condition is holding steady. "I'm doing good," he says. "It's status quo. I haven't gotten any worse. I can't probably lift more than thirty pounds or so. If I went to arm wrestle my eleven-year-old daughter, I couldn't beat her. But I can do all my daily life activities. I can live life every day."

On a recent checkup at Emory, Ted says, Dr. Glass told him something remarkable. "You're the first ALS patient I ever told this to," Glass said, "but right now you are not dying from ALS, you are living with it."

Ted looks back at the miracle he has undergone and wants to help others.

"I don't know why I was picked or why I was chosen," he says. "It's tough for me to think that I'm no more deserving than anyone else. But that kind of does drive my desire to help others because I feel like life is a gift you can't buy. So if I've been given this gift, how selfish is it of me to keep that gift to myself and not do something good with it.

"We all wonder sometimes what our purpose is," he says. "Maybe at the end of the day this is my purpose. The easy thing is to take your ball and go home. The hard thing is to do the work and try to make a difference even if it's an uphill battle and even if sometimes it impacts you physically. But I think my faith also tells me that my moral compass is if God gave you a gift; who am I to waste God's gift?

"I haven't seen the burning bush," he says, "but until I do I'm going to assume this is what He wants me to do."

Would he have the surgery again if his ALS symptoms began to return?

"That's not up to me," Ted says. "I wouldn't qualify for the trial anymore because it would be too long since my diagnosis, so if it gets to the point where I need it, if Right to Try doesn't exist, I'll be one of these people begging the FDA to give me a chance to live."

He says the government thinks it is protecting patients, but it's not.

"If you're on a plane that was crashing and there was a parachute, one parachute, and just because it didn't have a government stamp of approval on it, wouldn't you take your chance and try that parachute anyway? You would. If you looked at it and said, 'Oh, this thing's not certified, to heck with it, I guess I'll go down with the plane.' No, that's not what people would do. They'd take their chance with the parachute.

"I can go to Oregon and have the right to die, but it's not okay for me to try to save my life?" Ted says. "It just doesn't make sense."

Since word of his miraculous recovery spread, Ted has been inundated with requests for help from other patients.

"That's another reason why I'm so passionate," he says. "I get letters and emails—people begging me for their daughter, their spouse; what can you do to help me get into this trial? Obviously there's nothing I can do. And I also explained to them, you know, there's no guarantee that you'd get the result I got. And they say, 'Well, I know that, but I just want to try.' And it is heartbreaking some of these requests you get. And I just try to show them as much compassion as I can and give them as much support as I can."

He's also using the time he has been given to teach his kids important life lessons.

When he first got his diagnosis, he thought, "I could teach my kids how to deal with adversity, you know. Maybe when something bad happens in their life later on—because bad stuff happens—they can really be like, this is how my dad dealt with it. I wanted to show them that you have to hold your head high, and that was something that I wanted to impart to them."

Then, when he experienced his miraculous turnaround, the lesson changed.

"Now that I've been helped, I'm modeling the way for them that if you're given gifts, it's not just about the gift you received and, great, now you're happy, and you can be done. Now you have to see how you can help others. Whatever your gift or talent is you really have to see now how you can help others. And I try to impart that to them no matter what."

Recently, Ted was at the local hospital, visiting people from his church

"I was walking down the hall, and a lady comes out of her room and says, 'Are you Ted?' I said yes. She said, 'My name is Katie, we are connected on Facebook, and my husband, Bruce, has ALS.' She then told me that Bruce is in the hospital with pneumonia. I asked if I could meet Bruce. So she took me in their room and she told Bruce who I was and his eyes got big and he smiled. We talked for fifteen minutes and prayed together. His wife told me how hard they tried to get in the stem-cell trial but the timing didn't work out. They thanked me for all I do, which is so humbling because I am in awe of these patients dying without hope.

"It was a blessing to meet these people," he says. "We as a society need to do more than treat them as if their lives are a disposable commodity, and bicker over drug regulations for dying people."

DIEGO MORRIS RECENTLY WENT back to St. Jude Children's Research Hospital to have his prosthetic adjusted. Doctors at St. Jude had designed a special pediatric prosthetic that can be lengthened as he grows without additional surgeries.

"They put a ring around his leg; they put him under; they use heat and magnets and they pull the string and the prosthetic lengthens," his mom, Paulina, says.

The experience can be traumatic—imagine having your leg extended by an inch or more overnight. But two years after his treatment, Diego is doing great. Instead of going every three months for a body scan, he's able to go every six months now.

Mifamurtide—the drug the FDA denied him here at home—worked.

He's playing baseball again too. "He's a great athlete. He's not able to run, but that's really the only thing that slows him down," his father, Jason, says.

"We found him a super coach and team and it was very emotional for my husband and I to see him back on the pitching mound," says Paulina. "It's not the preference of the surgical artist, but our surgeon has I think three sons and he understands Diego's desire to be athletic."

As he resumes a normal teenage life, Diego is still fighting for the Right to Try. After his successful efforts to pass Right to Try in Arizona, he told us that he wanted to stay involved. So now he is helping make the case for Right to Try laws in other states.

"I am so fortunate to be cancer free," he says. "I want to help children who need medical treatment get the medicine they need at home. I want to help others."[3]

Diego and his family recently traveled to Oregon to talk with legislators and encourage them to pass Right to Try. He met members of the House Committee on Health Care and held a press conference in the state capitol with Representative Knute Buehler, an orthopedic surgeon who is the bill's principal sponsor.[4]

"I told them that I think Right to Try needs to pass because it's important that everyone has the ability to save their lives with experimental drugs and to save their families, and I think it's important that we get the drugs in the US when we need them," Diego says.

He's become a pretty effective advocate. Not long after Diego's visit, Right to Try passed the Oregon House by a unanimous 60 to 0 vote,[5] and the Senate by a unanimous 29 to 0 vote.

When Diego returned from his lobbying trip in Oregon, he was able to share his experiences with his social studies class. "It was fun telling my social studies teacher after the trip about the whole experience," Diego says, "because right now we're learning about the Arizona constitution and politics so it was fun telling about it."

He may have been the only kid in his class—or any eighth-grade class for that matter—who has actually changed the laws of his state.

His mom says the entire experience has transformed Diego.

"You never know how strong you are until you're faced with adversity," Paulina says. "And the opportunity to try and help others and make a difference and change a very stringent bureaucratic process here in the United States just has been amazing.

"In the United States we should be able to have options. We should be able to make informed decisions and have choices that we work in partnership with our doctor on in making informed choices, not just for ourselves but for our loved ones, for our children. This is the United States; we should be able to do that."

But to this day, Diego's government still has not approved the medication that helped save his life. And he is not the only one who needs it.

Some sixty-four hundred people in the United States have been diagnosed with osteosarcoma since the FDA rejected mifamurtide in 2007—about half of them children.[6] Not all of them can afford to move overseas to get the medication they need to save their lives as Diego did.

Why, Diego asks, should people have "to move five thousand miles away to receive treatment because our government could not approve a study after more than a decade? It's not right and nobody should have to go through the struggle of doing that. And not many people would even be able to do that. We were lucky to get the opportunity to go to London but not many people can just leave the country and go get a drug that should be approved but isn't."

Paulina's message to the FDA is simple:

"Listen up!" she says. "Listen up to what's happening around this country."

Right to Try has now passed in twenty-four states and counting, and the movement is showing no signs of slowing down.

"This is spreading like wildfire," she says. "You need to hear the changes that people want."

CHRIS GARABEDIAN, THE FORMER CEO of Sarepta, believes change is coming.

"What we've seen over the last couple of years is an increasing demand of patients across many disease areas of getting access to drugs that are in clinical development," he recently told the *Boston Business Journal*. "There's an increasing voice from the community [saying] that it is their right to get access to these investigational drugs, consistent with the Right to Try legislation."

Garabedian says, "The demand's not going away."

He's right. And neither is the Goldwater Institute . . . or Diego

Morris . . . or Ted Harada . . . or Frank Burroughs . . . or any of the countless heroes we've met who are fighting to get life-saving treatments to their fellow Americans before time runs out.

In chapter 1, Tracy Seckler, one of the Duchenne moms, compared the plight of their kids to the passengers on the *Titanic*. It's an apt analogy. As a society, we can and should debate the best ways to make better, stronger lifeboats. We can and should ensure the safety and reliability of lifeboats. We can and should figure out the best ways to pay for lifeboats and make sure we have more of them.

But there is no argument for *withholding* the lifeboats we do have from drowning kids.

Through the Right to Try movement, Americans are sending the powers that be an unmistakable message: Get those lifeboats in the water *right now*. We are not okay with letting those kids drown. Rescue those kids—and *then* figure out how to make better lifeboats.

And how are the opponents of Right to Try responding to this grassroots effort to rescue dying kids? With excuses: "We don't know if the lifeboats will work. . . . We don't want to give the drowning kids 'false hope.' . . . We don't have enough lifeboats for everyone, so we can't give them to anyone. . . . We don't know how to pay for the lifeboats. . . . It's not fair that the lifeboat manufacturers feel pressure to deploy them before they are ready. . . . We need to form a committee to decide who gets rescued and who doesn't. . . . We need to make sure there is a system in place to ensure people get in the lifeboats in an orderly fashion."

Good grief.

No wonder Right to Try is passing unanimously almost everywhere it comes up for a vote. On one hand, Americans see drowning kids. On the other, they see the government and the pharmaceutical industry making excuses for why we can't rescue them.

Does anyone doubt how this debate is going to play out?

The dying children will win.

This is why Richard Garr—who is quite explicit about the very real challenges in implementing these new laws—is on the Right to Try team. On the wall in his office, he keeps a reprint of a newspaper story about a young girl who had experimental gene therapy to treat a brain tumor. It failed and the girl died. He keeps the story, he says, to remind himself that "every day is the last day for somebody, someplace."[7]

We should all keep in mind the kids facing that last day as we debate these issues.

He's right. Boys with Duchenne . . . kids with osteosarcoma . . . moms with multiple myeloma . . . dads with Lou Gehrig's disease . . . young girls with brain tumors—they are all drowning right now. They don't have time to wait.

Let's get the lifeboats in the water.

# Acknowledgments

———

Let's be honest: I'm the mother of three toddlers. When a friend suggested that I write this book, the idea seemed preposterous. Where would I find the time?

My thanks go first to my collaborator, Marc Thiessen; and to the beloved friend who introduced us, Wynton Hall. Marc conducted dozens of interviews and flawlessly penned sentence after sentence to turn my ideas into this book. His buoyant humor made the work joyful, and the book possible.

For the conception of the Right to Try, I'm indebted to my friend Chuck Warren, who invited us to meet with the Cancer Treatment Centers of America to learn about the barriers to receiving life-saving treatments, and who challenged us to find a solution.

The Right to Try became our answer and was developed over several months by my extraordinarily talented colleagues, namely Kurt Altman, Clint Bolick, Starlee Coleman, Christina Corieri, Adi Dynar, and Christina Sandefur.

Through exceptional strategic acumen, Victor Riches drove the Right to Try in five states in rapid succession, passing the torch to Kurt

Altman, Craig Handzlik, and Michael Hunter, who made short work of taking the initiative to the next seventeen states.

We owe a great debt to our many on-the-ground partners, including the McLinn family, Linda Clark and Jehad Majed of PALS, Kelly Sawyer and her team at Change.org, Andi's Army and Michelle Wittenburg of the KK125 Ovarian Cancer Research Foundation, Lindsay Boyd and Justin Owen of the Beacon Center, Steve Buckstein of Cascade Policy Institute, Dr. Jameson Taylor of the Mississippi Center for Public Policy, Renae Cowley, and the State Policy Network.

Justin Lang, Dan Lips, Naomi Lopez-Bauman, and Christina Sandefur were the principal researchers on the book, cheerfully and meticulously slogging through reams of data to pinpoint truth. I'm also indebted to the UCLA law professor Eugene Volokh for his insightful review.

I'd also like to thank friends and colleagues who have contributed to this book in countless ways, including Annica Benning, Carol Carter, Matt Gallaher, Richard Garr, Michael Kelley, Beau and Amanda Law, Erik Merkow, Jon Riches, Stephanie Rugolo, Kris Schlott, Le Templar, Blake Wilson, Roger Zetah, and the Goldwater Institute's talented law clerks and interns.

The Goldwater Institute is funded entirely through donations, and the Right to Try simply would not exist without the thousands of committed men and women who generously support us. Thanks to Eric Crown, the Goldwater Institute board of directors, Tom and Sabina Sullivan, the JM Foundation, the Milbank Foundation, the Randolph Foundation, and Searle Freedom Trust for providing essential funding to turn the vision for the Right to Try into reality.

Thanks to the patients, family members, analysts, medical researchers, and physicians who shared their personal experiences for this book. I did my best to convey your voices and stories honestly and accurately and take full responsibility for any omissions or errors.

I've been blessed by many people in pursuit of this work but none so much as Norman McClelland, whose integrity and constancy provided light when dark skies appeared.

And finally, my gratitude to Adam Bellow, FE, for taking a chance on a new author, for patiently guiding the manuscript's development, and for what has become a bright friendship that I cherish.

# Notes

___

**INTRODUCTION**

1. Andrew von Eschenbach and Ralph Hall, "FDA Approvals Are a Matter of Life and Death," *Wall Street Journal*, June 17, 2012, accessed February 14, 2015, http://www.wsj.com/articles/SB10001424052702303753904577454163076760768.

2. "Debate over 'Right-to-Try' Laws," *The Diane Rehm Show*, National Public Radio, May 27, 2014, accessed March 14, 2015, http://thedianerehmshow.org/shows/2014-05-27/debate-over-right-try-laws.

3. "Expanded Access Submission Receipts Report (October 1, 2011–September 30, 2012)," US Food and Drug Administration, accessed March 4, 2015, http://www.fda.gov/downloads/Drugs/DevelopmentApprovalProcess/HowDrugsareDevelopedand Approved/DrugandBiologicApprovalReports/INDActivityReports/UCM390564.pdf.

4. "Cancer Facts & Figures 2012," American Cancer Society, accessed February 16, 2015, http://www.cancer.org/research/cancerfactsstatistics/cancerfactsfigures2012/.

5. Emily Rauhala, "North Korea Elections: A Sham Worth Studying," *Time*, March 10, 2014, accessed February 16, 2015, http://time.com/17720/north-korea-election-a-sham-worth-studying/.

6. "Arizona Terminal Patients' Right to Try Referendum, Proposition 303 (2014)," Ballotpedia, accessed March 3, 2015, http://ballotpedia.org/Arizona_Terminal_Patients%27_Right_to_Try_Referendum,_Proposition_303_%282014%29.

**CHAPTER 1: SOPHIE'S CHOICE**

1. Margaret Wahl, "Exon Skipping in DMD: What Is It and Whom Can It Help?" *Quest*, October 1, 2011, accessed February 3, 2015, http://quest.mda.org/article/exon-skipping-dmd-what-it-and-whom-can-it-help.

2. Balasubramanyam Seshan, "EU Patent Dispute Outcome Limits DMD Opportunity for AVI Biopharma," *International Business Times*, November 21, 2011, accessed February 23, 2015, http://www.ibtimes.com/eu-patent-dispute-outcome-limits-dmd-opportunity-avi-biopharma-372646.

3. Paul M. Barrett, "Moms, Regulators, Biotech Startups, and the Battle over a Potentially Life-Saving Drug," *Bloomberg Business*, October 30, 2014, accessed February 18, 2015, http://www.businessweek.com/printer/articles/233350-moms-regulators-biotech-startups-and-the-battle-over-a-potentially-life-saving-drug.

4. Luke Timmerman, "Profiles in Long-Termism: Sarepta Therapeutics CEO Chris Garabedian," *Xconomy*, June 10, 2013, accessed November 28, 2014, http://www.xconomy.com/national/2013/06/10/profiles-in-long-termism-sarepta-therapeutics-ceo-chris-garabedian/.

5. Ibid.

6. Don Seiffert, "Transcript of Interview with Former Sarepta CEO Chris Garabedian," *Boston Business Journal*, April 28, 2015, accessed May 3, 2015, http://www.bizjournals.com/boston/blog/bioflash/2015/04/transcript-of-interview-with-former-sarepta-ceo.html.

7. Timmerman, "Profiles in Long-Termism."

8. "Sarepta Therapeutics Announces Eteplirsen Meets Primary Endpoint of Increased Novel Dystrophin and Achieves Significant Clinical Benefit on 6-Minute Walk Test After 48 Weeks of Treatment in Phase IIb Study in Duchenne Muscular Dystrophy," Sarepta Therapeutics, October 3, 2013, accessed February 10, 2015, http://investorrelations.sarepta.com/phoenix.zhtml?c=64231&p=irol-newsArticle&ID=1741044.

9. "Sarepta Letter to Patient Community," Parent Project Muscular Dystrophy, accessed April 25, 2015, http://www.parentprojectmd.org/site/DocServer/Sarepta_Letter_to_Patient_Community_082812.pdf?docID=13303.

10. Seiffert, "Transcript of Interview with Former Sarepta CEO Chris Garabedian."

11. Barrett, "Moms, Regulators, Biotech Startups, and the Battle over a Potentially Life-Saving Drug."

12. Ibid.

13. Seiffert, "Transcript of Interview with Former Sarepta CEO Chris Garabedian."

14. "Sarepta Therapeutics Announces FDA Will Consider Accelerated Approval for Eteplirsen after Further Review of Data on Dystrophin and Clinical Outcomes," Sarepta Therapeutics, April 15, 2013, accessed May 12, 2015, http://investorrelations.sarepta.com/phoenix.zhtml?c=64231&p=irol-mediaPressArticle&ID=1806913.

15. "Sarepta Therapeutics Announces Plans to Submit New Drug Application to FDA for Eteplirsen for the Treatment of Duchenne Muscular Dystrophy in First Half of 2014," Sarepta Therapeutics, July 24, 2013, accessed May 12, 2015, http://investorrelations.sarepta.com/phoenix.zhtml?c=64231&p=irol-mediaPressArticle&ID=1840401.

16. Barrett, "Moms, Regulators, Biotech Startups, and the Battle over a Potentially Life-Saving Drug."

17. "Sarepta Therapeutics Announces FDA Considers NDA Filing for Eteplirsen Premature in Light of Recent Competitive Drug Failure and Recent DMD Natural History Data," Sarepta Therapeutics, November 12, 2013, accessed May 13, 2015, http://investorrelations.sarepta.com/phoenix.zhtml?c=64231&p=irol-mediaPressArticle&ID=1875187.

18. "Petition: Urge the FDA to Say Yes to Accelerated Approval for Safe, Effective Therapies for Children with Duchenne," The White House, accessed February 17, 2015, https://petitions.whitehouse.gov/petition/urge-fda-say-yes-accelerated-approval-safe-effective-therapies-children-duchenne.

19. Tracy Seckler, "Needless Delay for a Medicine That Could Save Kids' Lives," *Huffington Post*, March 5, 2014, accessed May 9, 2015, http://www.huffingtonpost.com/tracy-seckler/eteplirsen-duchenne_b_4904850.html.

20. "Sarepta Therapeutics Announces Plans to Submit New Drug Application to FDA for Eteplirsen for the Treatment of Duchenne Muscular Dystrophy by Year End 2014," Sarepta Therapeutics, April 21, 2014, accessed May 12, 2015, http://investorrelations.sarepta.com/phoenix.zhtml?c=64231&p=irol-mediaPressArticle&ID=1920025.

21. "Exon Skipping for Duchenne," Sarepta Therapeutics, accessed January 24, 2015, http://www.sarepta.com/pipeline/exon-skipping-duchenne.

## CHAPTER 2: FIVE THOUSAND MILES FOR A CURE

1. "What Are the Survival Rates for Osteosarcoma?" American Cancer Society, accessed December 9, 2014, http://www.cancer.org/cancer/osteosarcoma/detailedguide/osteosarcoma-survival-rates.

2. "Immune-Based Drug Approved in Europe for Pediatric Cancer Patients," MD Anderson Cancer Center, March 10, 2009, accessed February 5, 2015, http://www.mdanderson.org/newsroom/news-releases/2009/immune-based-drug-approved-in-europe-for-pediatric-cancer-patients.html.

3. E. S. Kleinerman, P. A. Meyers, C. L. Schwartz, et al., "Osteosarcoma: A Randomized, Prospective Trial of the Addition of Ifosfamide and/or Muramyl Tripeptide to Cisplatin, Doxorubicin, and High-Dose Methotrexate," *Journal of Clinical Oncology* 23 (2005): 2004, accessed May 13, 2015, doi: 10.1200/JCO.2005.06.031.

4. "The Journey of an Orphan Drug," *Children's Cancer Hospital Newsletter* (MD Anderson Cancer Center), Spring 2013, accessed April 25, 2015, http://www.mdanderson.org/publications/children-s-cancer-hospital-newsletter/issues/2013-spring/mepact.html.

5. Bonnie Mills, "Oncologic Drugs Advisory Committee on MTP for Osteosarcoma," presentation, Silver Spring, MD, May 9, 2007, accessed March 18, 2015, http://www.power show.com/view1/1f9c35-ZDc1Z/Oncologic_Drugs_Advisory_Committee_on_MTP_ for_Osteosarcoma_powerpoint_ppt_presentation.

6. "FDA Briefing Document—NDA 022092," Oncologic Drugs Advisory Committee, May 9, 2007, accessed March 15, 2015, http://www.fda.gov/ohrms/dockets/ac/07/ briefing/2007-4301b1-02-FDA-redacted.pdf.

7. Eugenie S. Kleinerman, "Oncologic Drugs Advisory Committee Hearing," Center for Drug Evaluation and Research, 57, May 9, 2007, accessed February 18, 2015, http://www .fda.gov/ohrms/dockets/ac/07/transcripts/2007-4301t1-Part1.pdf.

8. "IDM Pharma Receives Not Approvable Letter for Mifamurtide for Treatment of Osteosarcoma," *News Medical*, August 28, 2007, accessed January 29, 2015, http://www .news-medical.net/news/2007/08/28/29154.aspx.

9. "Mepact," European Medicines Agency, last modified January 10, 2013, accessed January 29, 2015, http://www.ema.europa.eu/ema/index.jsp?curl=pages/medicines/human/med icines/000802/human_med_000899.jsp&mid=WC0b01ac058001d124.

10. Lynne Taylor, "PAS Reverses NICE Rejection of Takeda's Mepact," *PharmaTimes*, October 27, 2011, accessed January 30, 2015, http://www.pharmatimes.com/Article/11-10-27/ PAS_reverses_NICE_rejection_of_Takeda_s_Mepact.aspx.

11. "Voters Approve Experimental-Drug Measure," KJZZ News, November 4, 2014, accessed April 21, 2015, http://kjzz.org/content/63525/voters-approve-experimental -drug-measure.

## CHAPTER 3: WHAT STEVE JOBS SAW

1. "Understanding Carcinoid Cancer," *Inside Mount Sinai*, December 21, 2008, accessed January 17, 2015, http://www.mountsinai.org/vgn_lnk/Regular%20Content/File/Faculty %20Profile%20Pdfs/MSN_inside_121508_Warner.pdf.

2. Walter Isaacson, *Steve Jobs* (New York: Simon & Schuster, 2011), 480.

3. "What Is an OctreoScan?" Carcinoid Cancer Foundation, accessed January 17, 2015, http://www.carcinoid.org/content/what-octreoscan.

4. D. J. Kwekkeboom, B. L. Kam, M. van Essen, et al., "Somatostatin Receptor-Based Imaging and Therapy of Gastroenteropancreatic Neuroendocrine Tumors," *Endocrine-Related Cancer* 17 (2010): R53–R73, accessed January 7, 2015, doi: 10.1677/erc-09-0078.

5. "What Is Peptide Receptor Radionuclide Therapy (PRRT)?" Society of Nuclear Medicine and Molecular Imaging, accessed March 20, 2014, http://snmmi.files.cms-plus.com/ docs/fact_sheets/PRRT_Final.pdf.

6. Lindsey Miller, "Ich Bin Eine Lebe," *I Am a Liver* (blog), May 24, 2013, accessed February 12, 2015, https://iamaliver.wordpress.com/2013/05/24/ich-bin-eine-lebe/.

7. Lindsey Miller, "Crowdfunding My Cancer Care," *Huffington Post*, April 3, 2014, accessed

February 13, 2015, http://www.huffingtonpost.com/lindsey-miller/crowdfunding-for-my-medic_b_5073305.html.

8. Jaclyn Cosgrove, "Oklahoma Vietnam Veteran with Cancer Asks Why VA Won't Cover His Care," *Daily Oklahoman*, June 22, 2014, accessed May 1, 2015, http://newsok.com/oklahoma-vietnam-veteran-with-cancer-asks-why-va-wont-cover-his-care/article/4949250/?page=1.

9. "Netter-1 Study," Advanced Accelerator Applications, accessed March 21, 2015, http://www.adacap.com/netter-1/.

10. D. Wild, M. Fani, R. Fischer, et al., "Comparison of Somatostatin Receptor Agonist and Antagonist for Peptide Receptor Radionuclide Therapy: A Pilot Study," *Journal of Nuclear Medicine* 55 (2014): 1248–52, accessed January 9, 2015, doi: 10.2967/jnumed.114.138834.

11. Marsha Shuler, "'Dallas Buyers Club' Bill Signed into Law in La.," *The Advocate,* June 2, 2014, accessed April 5, 2015, http://theadvocate.com/news/9317769-123/dallas-buyers-club-bill-signed.

## CHAPTER 4: MAKING MEDICAL MIRACLES

1. "Serendipity," Mayo Clinic, accessed February 26, 2015, http://www.mayoclinic.org/giving-to-mayo-clinic/your-impact/features-stories/serendipity.

2. Ibid.

3. Lindsey Seavert, "Mayo Clinic Trial: Massive Measles Vaccine Attacks Blood Cancer," *KARE* 11, May 15, 2014, accessed May 13, 2015, http://www.kare11.com/story/news/health/2014/05/14/mayo-clinic-trial-measles-vaccine-multiple-myeloma/9101893/.

4. Lizzy Smith, "An Interview with Stacy Erholtz on Getting the Measles Vaccine & Participating in Clinical Trials," *Myeloma Crowd*, October 22, 2014, accessed January 27, 2015, http://www.myelomacrowd.org/interview-stacy-erholtz-getting-measles-vaccine-participating-clinical-trials/.

5. "Serendipity," Mayo Clinic.

6. Dan Browning, "Mayo Clinic Trial: Massive Blast of Measles Vaccine Wipes Out Cancer," *Minneapolis Star Tribune*, December 18, 2014, accessed March 9, 2015, http://www.startribune.com/no-4-massive-blast-of-measles-vaccine-wipes-out-cancer-in-mayo-clinic-trial/259155541/.

7. Lindsey Bever, "Woman's Cancer Killed by Measles Virus in Unprecedented Trial," *Washington Post*, May 15, 2014, accessed March 28, 2015, http://www.washingtonpost.com/news/morning-mix/wp/2014/05/15/womans-cancer-killed-by-measles-virus-in-unprecedented-trial/.

8. Lecia Bushak, "Measles Virus Cures Cancer in Woman with Multiple Myeloma; Stacy Erholtz Now Fundraising More Research," *Medical Daily*, September 12, 2014, accessed March 12, 2015, http://www.medicaldaily.com/measles-virus

-cures-cancer-woman-multiple-myeloma-stacy-erholtz-now-fundraising-more
-302850.

9. Jacque Wilson and William Hudson, "Measles Virus Used to Put Woman's Cancer into Remission," CNN, May 18, 2014, accessed April 17, 2015, http://www.cnn.com/2014/05/15/health/measles-cancer-remission/.

10. Scott Pelley, "Killing Cancer," *60 Minutes*, CBS, aired March 29, 2015, accessed March 30, 2015, http://www.cbsnews.com/news/polio-cancer-treatment-duke-university-60-minutes-scott-pelley/.

11. Ibid.

12. Ibid.

13. "Providence Brain and Cancer Experts Begin First-in-World Novel Brain Tumor Vaccine Research Trial," *Providence Health & Services*, May 5, 2014, accessed April 2, 2015, http://oregon.providence.org/news-and-events/news/2014/05/providence-brain-and-cancer-experts-begin-first-in-world-novel-brain-tumor-vaccine-research-trial/.

14. Ibid.

15. Shannon O. Wells, "'Luckiest Guy' Gets a New Lease on Life," *Beaverton Valley Times*, July 2, 2014, accessed April 4, 2015, http://www.pamplinmedia.com/bvt/15-news/226045-88134-luckiest-guy-gets-a-new-lease-on-life.

16. Browning, "Mayo Clinic Trial."

17. "Fire with Fire—Ross Kauffman—GE Focus Forward," YouTube video, 3:39, posted by "General Electric," May 5, 2013, https://www.youtube.com/watch?v=h6SzI2ZfPd4.

18. "Childhood Acute Lymphoblastic Leukemia Treatment—for Health Professionals (PDQ®)," National Cancer Institute, last modified May 20, 2015, accessed May 26, 2015, http://www.cancer.gov/types/leukemia/hp/child-all-treatment-pdq#section/all.

19. "Fire with Fire—Ross Kauffman—GE Focus Forward," YouTube video.

20. Matthew Herper, "Is This How We'll Cure Cancer?" *Forbes*, May 7, 2014, accessed May 20, 2015, http://www.forbes.com/sites/matthewherper/2014/05/07/is-this-how-well-cure-cancer/.

21. Ibid.

22. "How Many People Get Acute Lymphocytic Leukemia?," American Cancer Society, last modified January 12, 2015, accessed April 15, 2015, http://www.cancer.org/cancer/leukemia-acutelymphocyticallinadults/overviewguide/leukemia-all-overview-key-statistics.

23. "Glioblastoma Multiforme," *American Association of Neurological Surgeons*, March 2015, accessed May 6, 2015, http://www.aans.org/Patient%20Information/Conditions%20and%20Treatments/Glioblastoma%20Multiforme.aspx.

24. "How Many People Get Multiple Myeloma?" American Cancer Society, last modified June 19, 2014, accessed April 15, 2015, http://www.cancer.org/cancer/multiplemyeloma/overviewguide/multiple-myeloma-overview-key-statistics.

25. "Fight to Live," *Gravitas Ventures*, directed by Barbara Kopple (2014).

26. "Dr. John C. Bell," Ottawa Hospital Research Institute, accessed April 16, 2015, http://www.ohri.ca/corporate/jbell.asp.

27. John C. Bell, Caroline J. Breitbach, et al., "Intravenous Delivery of a Multi-Mechanistic Cancer-Targeted Oncolytic Poxvirus in Humans," *Nature* 477 (2011): 99–102, accessed May 1, 2015, doi:10.1038/nature10358.

## CHAPTER 5: INSIDE MAN

1. Kathleen Doheny, "When Depression Becomes Deadly," WebMD, August 14, 2014, accessed March 3, 2015, http://www.webmd.com/depression/news/20140812/depression-deadly.

2. "FDA Approves Neuralstem to Treat Final Cohort in NSI-189 Phase Ib Trial in Major Depressive Disorder," Neuralstem Inc., accessed February 21, 2015, http://investor.neuralstem.com/2013-04-22-FDA-Approves-Neuralstem-To-Treat-Final-Cohort-In-NSI-189-Phase-Ib-Trial-In-Major-Depressive-Disorder.

3. David Frey, "A Better Pill to Swallow," *Bethesda Magazine*, November-December 2013, accessed March 2, 2015, http://www.bethesdamagazine.com/Bethesda-Magazine/November-December-2013/NSI-189/.

4. Kim Kozlowski, "UM Researcher Uses Stem Cells to Fight Alzheimer's," *Detroit News*, November 11, 2014, accessed April 25, 2015, http://www.detroitnews.com/story/news/local/michigan/2014/11/11/um-researcher-uses-stem-cells-fight-alzheimers/18895621/.

5. Richard Garr, "Post: December 2, 2013," Neuralstem Inc. blog, December 2, 2013, accessed December 14, 2014, http://www.neuralstem.com/neuralstem-ceo-blog/208-every-man-gotta-right-to-decide-his-own-destiny.

6. Andrew Pollack, "Ebola Therapy from an Obscure Biotech Firm Is Hurried Along," *New York Times*, August 6, 2014, accessed February 25, 2015, http://www.nytimes.com/2014/08/07/business/an-obscure-biotech-firm-hurries-ebola-treatment.html.

7. Lenny Bernstein and Brady Dennis, "Small Drugmakers Try to Scale Up to Meet Ebola Crisis," *Washington Post*, October 9, 2014, accessed January 9, 2015, http://www.washingtonpost.com/national/health-science/2014/10/09/a594dec2-4fee-11e4-babe-e91da079cb8a_story.html.

8. Sheri Fink and Rick Gladstone, "Two Vaccines to Protect Against Ebola Could Be Available Within Weeks," *New York Times*, September 5, 2014, accessed January 11, 2015, http://www.nytimes.com/2014/09/06/world/africa/ebola-vaccine-could-be-ready-by-november-who-says.html.

9. Richard Garr, "The FDA Is Not the Enemy," *The Chairman's Blog*, June 9, 2014, accessed March 2, 2015, http://www.thechairmansblog.com/neuralstem/richard-garr/fda-enemy/.

10. Amy Dockser Marcus, "Frustrated ALS Patients Concoct Their Own Drug," *Wall Street Journal*, April 15, 2012, accessed January 7, 2015, http://www.wsj.com/articles/SB10001424052702304818404577345953943484054.

**CHAPTER 6: WE ARE THE 99 PERCENT**

1. Linda Carroll, "Mom's Heartache: Two Sons Have Deadly Disease, but Only One Can Get 'Miracle Drug,'" NBC News, May 27, 2013, accessed May 1, 2015, http://www.today .com/health/moms-heartache-two-sons-have-deadly-disease-only-one-can-6C10077829.

2. Kylee Wierks, "Boy with Fatal Condition Gets Dream Job with IFD," Fox 59, December 24, 2014, accessed May 1, 2015, http://fox59.com/2014/12/24/boy-with -fatal-condition-to-interview-for-dream-job-with-ifd/.

3. Derrik Thomas, "5-Year-Old Gets Wish, 'Hired' by IFD," RTV6 ABC, December 25, 2014, accessed May 1, 2015, http://www.theindychannel.com/news/local-news/ watch-5-year-old-gets-wish-hired-by-ifd.

4. Matt Smith, "Five-Year-Old Indiana Boy to Lawmakers: 'Please Say Yes' to Right to Try Bill," Fox 59, March 4, 2015, accessed May 1, 2015, http://fox59.com/2015/03/04/ indiana-boy-to-lawmakers-please-say-yes-to-right-to-try-bill/.

5. Jessica Firger, "Indiana Governor Signs 'Right to Try' Drug Law," CBS News, March 24, 2015, accessed May 2, 2015, http://www.cbsnews.com/news/ indiana-governor-signs-right-to-try-drug-law/.

6. "The Little Boy Behind Indiana's 'Right to Try' Bill," CBS News, March 25, 2015, accessed May 3, 2015, http://www.cbsnews.com/news/jordan-mclinn-5-year-old-face -behind-indiana-right-to-try-bill-muscular-dystrophy/.

7. Kevin Rader, "Five-Year-Old Hero's Fight Begins as Pence Signs 'Right to Try' Bill," WTHR, March 24, 2015, accessed May 3, 2015, http://www.wthr.com/story/28598710/ pence-set-to-sign-right-to-try-bill.

8. "Save Locky's Dad," YouTube video, 3:25, posted by "Savelockys Dadnick," August 28, 2013, https://www.youtube.com/watch?v=3teA62o5eLY.

9. Sydney Lupkin, "Dad Pleading for Unapproved Cancer Drug Dies," ABC News, November 25, 2013, accessed February 26, 2015, http://abcnews.go.com/Health/ dad-pleading-unapproved-cancer-drug-dies/story?id=21004482&singlePage=true.

10. Save Locky's Dad Facebook page, last modified November 24, 2013, accessed May 2, 2015, https://www.facebook.com/savelockysdad/photos/a.213259775503468 .1073741830.208927279270051/237716026391176/.

11. Kurtis Lee, "'Right to Try' Aims to Limit Bureaucracy for Colorado's Terminally Ill," *Denver Post*, April 1, 2014, accessed May 2, 2015, http://www.denverpost.com/politics/ ci_25463368/right-try-aims-limit-bureaucracy-colorados-terminally-ill.

12. Kristen Wyatt, "Governor Signs Ginal's 'Right to Try' Bill," *Coloradoan*, May 17, 2014, accessed May 2, 2015, http://www.coloradoan.com/story/news/local/2014/05/17/ gov-signs-ginals-right-try-bill/9232409/.

13. Edie Bacon, "My Life's Not FDA-Approved," *Wall Street Journal*, November 29, 2002, accessed May 1, 2015, http://www.wsj.com/articles/SB1038535925179938868.

14. "Yondelis," European Medicines Agency, last modified September 10, 2012, accessed

May 4, 2015, http://www.ema.europa.eu/ema/index.jsp?curl=pages/medicines/human/medicines/000773/human_med_001165.jsp.

15. "U.S. FDA Grants Priority Review for Yondelis (Trabectedin) for the Treatment of Patients with Advanced Soft Tissue Sarcoma," Drugs.com, February 3, 2015, accessed May 2, 2014, http://www.drugs.com/nda/yondelis_150203.html.

16. Kristina Brogan, interviewed by Stephen Fee, "'Right to Try' Law Gives Terminal Patients Access to Drugs Not Approved by FDA," *PBS News Hour*, June 21, 2014, accessed April 29, 2015, http://www.pbs.org/newshour/bb/right-try-law-gives-terminal-patients-access-non-fda-approved-drugs/.

17. Mike Sherry, "Missouri Becomes Third State to Enact 'Right to Try' Drug Therapy Law," *KCPT*, July 15, 2014, accessed December 19, 2014, http://kcpt.org/health/missouri-state-enact-right-try-drug-therapy-law/.

18. Nick Swedberg, "'Right to Try' Medical Measure Sent to Illinois Governor," Associated Press, May 19, 2015, accessed May 25, 2015, http://www.nwherald.com/2015/05/19/right-to-try-medical-measure-sent-to-illinois-governor/aa30hvt/.

19. "Connelly and Harris Aim to Give Terminal Patients Options," Illinois Senate GOP, January 30, 2015, accessed March 15, 2015, http://senategop.state.il.us/News/Recent News/TabId/121/p/24811/v/2000/connelly-and-harris-aim-to-give-terminal-patients-options.aspx#sthash.TrEMtw6m.dpuf.

20. Andi's Army Facebook page, accessed March 15, 2015, https://www.facebook.com/OfficialAndisArmy.

21. "BioMarin Pharmaceutical: Give Andrea Sloan (@andi_sloan) Access to the Cancer Drug That Could Save Her Life," Change.org, accessed April 9, 2015, https://www.change.org/p/biomarin-pharmaceutical-give-andrea-sloan-andi-sloan-access-to-the-cancer-drug-that-could-save-her-life.

22. Shannon Wolfson, "Andrea Sloan Pleads with BioMarin CEO," KXAN-TV, September 25, 2013, accessed March 15, 2015, http://kxan.com/2013/09/25/andrea-sloan-pleads-biomarin-ceo/.

23. Jason Cherkis, "Andrea Sloan Wins Big Victory in Quest for Cancer Drug," *Huffington Post*, October 3, 2013, accessed March 15, 2015, http://www.huffingtonpost.com/2013/10/03/andrea-sloan-victory-drug_n_4039633.html.

24. Todd Ackerman, "Texas Poised to Pass Right-to-Try Legislation," *Houston Chronicle*, May 9, 2015, accessed May 6, 2015, http://www.houstonchronicle.com/news/health/article/Texas-poised-to-pass-right-to-try-legislation-6253623.php.

25. "Joshua Hardy," CaringBridge, accessed May 7, 2015, http://www.caringbridge.org/visit/joshuahardy/mystory.

26. Robert Griffin III, Twitter post, March 10, 2014, 9:47 a.m., https://twitter.com/rgiii/status/443065599863033857.

27. Elizabeth Cohen, "Company Denies Drug to Dying Child," CNN, March 11, 2014, accessed December 17, 2014, http://www.cnn.com/2014/03/10/health/cohen-josh/.

28. "Company Denies Drug to 7-Year-Old Boy Struggling against Curable Virus," Fox News, March 10, 2014, accessed May 7, 2015, http://insider.foxnews.com/2014/03/10/drug-maker-chimerix-refuses-release-drug-7-year-old-josh-hardy-struggles-against-curable.

29. "Charity Offers to Pay for 7-Year-Old's Lifesaving Treatment; Drug Maker Still Refuses," Fox News, March 11, 2014, accessed May 7, 2015, http://www.foxnews.com/health/2014/03/11/charity-offers-to-pay-for-7-year-old-lifesaving-treatment-drug-maker-still/.

30. "Chimerix Board Member Blames FDA for 7-Year-Old Josh Hardy's Plight," Fox News, March 12, 2014, accessed May 4, 2015, http://www.foxnews.com/health/2014/03/12/chimerix-board-member-blames-fda-for-7-year-old-josh-hardys-plight/.

31. Doreen Gentzler, "#SaveJosh: With Help of Social Media, Va. Boy Gets Experimental Drug," NBC Washington, February 20, 2015, accessed May 7, 2015, http://www.nbcwashington.com/news/local/Josh-Hardy-8-Year-Old-Virginia-Boy-Thanks-Social-Media-After-Experimental-Drug-292771561.html.

32. "Lawmakers and Parents Advocate for Right to Try Legislation," NBC 29, February 23, 2015, accessed April 12, 2015, http://www.nbc29.com/story/28177028/lawmakers-and-parents-advocate-for-right-to-try-legislation.

33. Victoria Zawitkowski, "Virginia Lawmakers Make Final Push for Passage of 'Josh Hardy' Bill," February 23, 2015, accessed May 7, 2015, *Free Lance-Star*, http://www.fredericksburg.com/news/virginia/virginia-lawmakers-make-final-push-for-passage-of-josh-hardy/article_df418a48-bba1-11e4-84f1-7f77ffb94cdc.html.

34. Compassionate Use of Investigational New Drugs: Is the Current Process Effective? Hearing Before the Committee on Government Reform, House of Representatives, 107th Cong. 37-38 (2001) (Testimony of Frank Burroughs).

35. "House, Senate Leaders Announce Agreement on Right to Try Legislation," *Augusta Free Press*, February 23, 2015, accessed March 26, 2015, http://augustafreepress.com/house-senate-leaders-announce-agreement-on-right-to-try-legislation/.

36. Robyn Sidersky, "Governor Signs 'Right to Try' Bill Inspired by Josh Hardy," *Free Lance-Star*, March 27, 2015, accessed May 8, 2015, http://www.fredericksburg.com/news/local/fredericksburg/governor-signs-right-to-try-bill-inspired-by-josh-hardy/article_978ee80e-d3ec-11e4-8beb-271596aa66ff.html.

37. "Lawmakers and Parents Advocate for Right to Try Legislation," NBC29 WVIR-TV, last modified February 23, 2015, accessed May 8, 2015, http://www.nbc29.com/story/28177028/lawmakers-and-parents-advocate-for-right-to-try-legislation.

38. Robin Erb, "Michigan Senate Panel OKs Bill Offering Wider Access to Experimental Drugs," *Detroit Free Press*, July 16, 2014, accessed May 8, 2015, http://archive.freep.com/article/20140716/NEWS06/307160136/experimental-medications-Michigan-bill.

39. Steve Carmody, "Michigan Will Give Terminally Ill Patients the Right to Try Experimental Treatments," Michigan Radio, October 17, 2014, accessed May 8, 2015,

http://michiganradio.org/post/michigan-will-give-terminally-ill-patients-right-try
-experimental-treatments.

40. Abby Simons, "For Rep. Nick Zerwas, 'Right to Try' Legislation Is from the Heart," *StarTribune*, May 2, 2015, accessed May 8, 2015, http://www.startribune.com/ for-rep-nick-zerwas-right-to-try-legislation-is-from-the-heart/302311191/.

41. "Governor Bentley Signs 'Gabe's Right to Try' Act into Law" Office of Alabama Governor Robert J. Bentley, June 3, 2015, accessed June 8, 2015, http://governor.alabama.gov/ newsroom/2015/06/governor-bentley-signs-gabes-right-try-act-law/.

42. Patrick Springer, "N.D. Family Fighting Rare Disease Pleads for 'Right to Try' Law to Enable Experimental Drug," WDAZ-8 ABC News, March 11, 2015, accessed May 8, 2015, http://www.wdaz.com/news/north-dakota/3697527-nd-family-fighting-rare -disease-pleads-right-try-law-enable-experimental.

43. Courtney Ann Jackson, "Right to Try Act Could Bring Needed Hope for Terminally Ill Patients," *Mississippi News Now*, January 29, 2016, accessed May 3, 2015, http:// www.msnewsnow.com/story/27978780/right-to-try-act-could-bring-needed-hope-for -terminally-ill-patients.

## CHAPTER 7: COMPASSIONATE USE

1. Mike Sherry, "Missouri Becomes Third State to Enact 'Right to Try' Drug Therapy Law," KCPT, July 15, 2014, accessed December 19, 2014, http://kcpt.org/health/ missouri-state-enact-right-try-drug-therapy-law/.

2. "Give My Wife a Chance against Cancer: Please Grant Compassionate Use of MK-3475 for Mikaela Right Away," Change.org, accessed May 9, 2015, https://www.change.org/p/ merck-please-grant-compassionate-use-of-mk-3475-for-mikaela-right-away.

3. "Dying Woman's Hope Buoyed by Campaign for Experimental Drug," ABC News, March 27, 2014, accessed April 8, 2015, http://abcnews.go.com/blogs/headlines/2014/03/ dying-womans-hope-buoyed-by-campaign-for-experimental-drug/.

4. Matthew Herper, "Merck Cancer Drug Shines Against Skin, Lung Cancer," *Forbes*, April 19, 2015, accessed May 27, 2015, http://www.forbes.com/sites/matthewherper/2015/04/19/ merck-cancer-drug-shines-against-skin-lung-cancer/.

5. "How About a 'Kianna's Law'?" *Wall Street Journal*, March 24, 2005, accessed May 5, 2015, http://www.wsj.com/articles/SB111163190273988429.

6. Jerome Groopman, "The Right to a Trial," *New Yorker*, December 18, 2006, accessed January 8, 2015, http://www.newyorker.com/magazine/2006/12/18/the-right -to-a-trial.

7. Right to Try: Colorado HB14-281, Hearing Before the House Health, Insurance & Environment Committee, Colorado General Assembly, March 13, 2014 (Testimony of Josh Gordon), http://azbio.tv/video/9775c0b16bbe4667a6dd34c4e1d00883.

8. Compassionate Use of Investigational New Drugs: Is the Current Process Effective?

Hearing Before the Committee on Government Reform, House of Representatives, 107th Cong. 37-38 (2001) (Testimony of Frank Burroughs).

9. US Food and Drug Administration, "Expanded Access INDs and Protocols" accessed April 6, 2015, http://www.fda.gov/Drugs/DevelopmentApprovalProcess/HowDrugs areDevelopedandApproved/DrugandBiologicApprovalReports/INDActivityReports/ ucm373560.htm.

10. "Cancer Facts & Figures 2015," American Cancer Society, accessed January 17, 2015, http://www.cancer.org/research/cancerfactsstatistics/cancerfactsfigures2015/index.

11. Institute of Medicine (US) Forum on Drug Discovery, Development, and Translation, "Transforming Clinical Research in the United States: Challenges and Opportunities: Workshop Summary," Washington, DC: National Academies Press (US), 2010, 6, Clinical Trials in Cancer. Available from: http://www.ncbi.nlm.nih.gov/books/NBK50895/.

12. Emil J. Freireich, "Should Terminally Ill Patients Have the Right to Take Drugs That Pass Phase I Testing? Yes." *British Medical Journal* 335 (2007): 478, accessed March 1, 2015, doi:10.1136/bmj.39244.451192.AD.

13. "Impact Report Summary: Growing Protocol Design Complexity Stresses Investigators, Volunteers," Tufts Center for the Study of Drug Development, January 2008, accessed February 25, 2015, http://csdd.tufts.edu/files/uploads/jan-feb_impact_report_summary.pdf.

14. "Texas Woman with Cancer Pressuring Experimental Drug Maker for 'Compassionate' Access," CBS News, September 10, 2013, accessed March 3, 2015, http://www.cbsnews .com/news/texas-woman-with-cancer-pressuring-experimental-drug-maker-for -compassionate-access/.

15. Freireich, "Should Terminally Ill Patients Have the Right."

16. "Poll: How Doctors Feel about Compassionate Use," SERMO, February 23, 2015, accessed March 28, 2015, http://blog.sermo.com/2015/02/23/poll-doctors-feel-compassionate-use/.

17. Sam Kazman, "A National Survey of Orthopedic Surgeons Regarding the Food and Drug Administration and the Availability of New Therapies," Competitive Enterprise Institute, January 30, 2007, accessed February 19, 2015, http://cei.org/sites/default/files/ The%20Polling%20Company%20-%20A%20National%20Survey%20of%20Ortho pedic%20Surgeons%20Regarding%20the%20Food%20and%20Drug%20Administra tion%20and%20the%20Availability%20of%20New%20Therapies.pdf.

18. "Early Access Programs: Points to Consider," Biotechnology Industry Organization's Board Standing Committee on Bioethics, April 16, 2010, accessed February 20, 2015, https://www.bio.org/sites/default/files/20100416.pdf.

19. Michael Rosenblatt and Bruce Kuhlik, "Principles and Challenges in Access to Experimental Medicines," *JAMA: The Journal of the American Medical Association* 313 (2015): 2023–24, accessed June 3, 2015. doi:10.1001/jama.2015.4135.

20. Frank Young, interview with Judy Woodruff, *The MacNeil/Lehrer NewsHour*, PBS, February 16, 1988.

21. Philip M. Boffey, "Campaign to Find Drugs for Fighting AIDS Is Intensified," *New York Times*, February 15, 1988, accessed May 1, 2015, http://www.nytimes.com/1988/02/15/us/campaign-to-find-drugs-for-fighting-aids-is-intensified.html.

22. "Drugs to Fight AIDS Given Top Priority at FDA," *Associated Press*, January 30, 1988, accessed May 1, 2015, http://articles.latimes.com/1988-01-30/news/mn-10189_1_top-priority.

23. Rebecca Kolberg, "Protesters Demanding Faster Access to AIDS Treatments Were Arrested," United Press International, October 11, 1988, accessed May 13, 2015, http://www.upi.com/Archives/1988/10/11/Protesters-demanding-faster-access-to-AIDS-treatments-were-arrested/7539592545600/.

24. Steve Usdin, "States' Rights," *BioCentury*, June 30, 2014, accessed March 15, 2015, http://www.biocentury.com/biotech-pharma-news/politics/2014-06-30/as-right-to-try-landscape-expands-in-us-so-does-debate-on-laws-effect-a1.

25. Kathy Wren, "Faster Approval of New Medical Products Heightens Uncertainty over Risks," American Association for the Advancement of Science, July 7, 2014, accessed March 22, 2015, http://www.aaas.org/news/faster-approval-new-medical-products-heightens-uncertainty-over-risks.

26. Margaret A. Hamburg, "A Pivotal Moment for the Treatment of Rare Diseases," speech delivered at the NORD Rare Diseases and Orphan Products Breakthrough Summit, Alexandria, VA, October 22, 2014.

27. Douglas Crimp, "Before Occupy: How AIDS Activists Seized Control of the FDA in 1988," *The Atlantic*, December 6, 2011, accessed February 18, 2015, http://www.theatlantic.com/health/archive/2011/12/before-occupy-how-aids-activists-seized-control-of-the-fda-in-1988/249302/.

28. Gina Kolata, "Patients Going Underground to Buy Experimental Drugs," *New York Times*, November 4, 1991, accessed February 4, 2015, http://www.nytimes.com/1991/11/04/us/patients-going-underground-to-buy-experimental-drugs.html.

29. "Debate over 'Right-to-Try' Laws," *The Diane Rehm Show*, National Public Radio, May 27, 2014, accessed March 14, 2015, http://thedianerehmshow.org/shows/2014-05-27/debate-over-right-try-laws.

30. Peter Lurie, "A Big Step to Help the Patients Most in Need," *FDA Voice*, February 4, 2015, accessed February 26, 2015, http://blogs.fda.gov/fdavoice/index.php/2015/02/a-big-step-to-help-the-patients-most-in-need/.

31. "Debate over 'Right-to-Try' Laws," *The Diane Rehm Show*.

32. Arthur Caplan and Kenneth Moch, "Rescue Me: The Challenge of Compassionate Use in the Social Media Era," *Health Affairs*, August 27, 2014, accessed January 8, 2015, http://healthaffairs.org/blog/2014/08/27/rescue-me-the-challenge-of-compassionate-use-in-the-social-media-era/.

33. "Fight to Live," *Gravitas Ventures*, directed by Barbara Kopple (2014).

34. Crimp, "Before Occupy."

35. "How About a 'Kianna's Law'?" *Wall Street Journal*.

36. Scott Gottlieb, "The FDA Is Evading the Law," *Wall Street Journal*, December 23, 2010, accessed January 22, 2015, http://www.wsj.com/articles/SB1000142405274870403480457 6025981869663212.

37. "Kianna's Law," *Wall Street Journal*, November 15, 2005, accessed January 17, 2015, http://www.wsj.com/articles/SB113202333332497225.

38. C. Bélorgey, "Temporary Authorisations for Use (ATU)," Agence Française de Sécurité Sanitaire des Produits de Santé, June 2011, accessed April 18, 2015, http://agence-tst .ansm.sante.fr/html/pdf/5/atu_eng.pdf.

## CHAPTER 8: WOULD YOU USE A FIFTEEN-YEAR-OLD CELL PHONE?

1. Margaret A. Hamburg, Remarks at the National Press Club Speaker Luncheon, October 6, 2010, transcript accessed February 3, 2015, http://www.fda.gov/NewsEvents/ Speeches/ucm229195.htm.

2. Executive Office of the President and President's Council of Advisors on Science and Technology, "Report to the President on Propelling Innovation in Drug Discovery, Development, and Evaluation," September 2012, accessed April 11, 2015, https://www .whitehouse.gov/sites/default/files/microsites/ostp/pcast-fda-final.pdf.

3. Janet Woodcock and Karen Midthun, "US Can Continue to Lead in Drug Innovation," *The Hill*, March 10, 2015, accessed April 18, 2015, http://thehill.com/opinion/ op-ed/235278-us-can-continue-to-lead-in-drug-innovation.

4. US Food and Drug Administration, Center for Drug Evaluation and Research, *Novel New Drugs 2014 Summary*, January 2015, accessed April 23, 2015, http://www.fda.gov/ downloads/Drugs/DevelopmentApprovalProcess/DrugInnovation/UCM430299.pdf.

5. Scott Gottlieb, "Changing the FDA's Culture," *National Affairs*, Summer 2012, accessed April 20, 2015, http://www.nationalaffairs.com/publications/detail/changing-the -fdas-culture.

6. "Enzyme Replacement Drug Found to Be Effective Treatment for Hunter Syndrome," University of North Carolina School of Medicine, August 21, 2006, accessed January 19, 2015, http://www.sciencedaily.com/releases/2006/08/060819115541.htm.

7. US Food and Drug Administration, "FDA Approves First Treatment for Hunter Syndrome," news release, July 24, 2006, accessed April 19, 2015, http://www.fda.gov/News Events/Newsroom/PressAnnouncements/2006/ucm108699.htm.

8. Kenneth A. Getz and Kenneth I. Kaitin, "Why Is the Pharmaceutical and Biotechnology Industry Struggling?" in *Re-Engineering Clinical Trials*, ed. Peter Schuler and Brendan M. Buckley (London: Academic Press, 2015), 9.

9. Ibid., 10–11.

10. "What Is Idiopathic Pulmonary Fibrosis?" National Heart, Lung, and Blood Institute,

last modified September 20, 2011, accessed April 18, 2015, http://www.nhlbi.nih.gov/health/health-topics/topics/ipf.

11. Andrew Pollack, "InterMune Lung Drug Is Successful in New Trial," *New York Times*, February 25, 2014, accessed April 19, 2015, http://www.nytimes.com/2014/02/26/business/intermune-reports-successful-trial-for-lung-disease-drug.html.

12. Andrew Pollack, "F.D.A. Rejects InterMune's Drug for Fatal Lung Disease," *New York Times*, May 4, 2010, accessed April 19, 2015, http://www.nytimes.com/2010/05/05/business/05lung.html.

13. US Food and Drug Administration, "FDA Approves Esbriet to Treat Idiopathic Pulmonary Fibrosis," news release, October 15, 2014, accessed April 21, 2015, http://www.fda.gov/NewsEvents/Newsroom/PressAnnouncements/ucm418991.htm.

14. Joyce Frieden, "FDA Nixes Pirfenidone for Now, Wants New Trial," *MedPage Today*, May 5, 2010, accessed April 20, 2015, http://www.medpagetoday.com/PublicHealthPolicy/FDAGeneral/19933.

15. "InterMune Receives FDA Breakthrough Therapy Designation for Pirfenidone, an Investigational Treatment for IPF," Coalition for Pulmonary Fibrosis, accessed April 21, 2015, http://www.coalitionforpf.org/2014/07/17/ntermune-receives-fda-breakthrough-therapy-designation-for-pirfenidone-an-investigational-treatment-for-ipf/.

16. "InterMune Reports Japanese Regulatory Approval of Pirfenidone in IPF," Coalition for Pulmonary Fibrosis, accessed April 21, 2015, http://www.coalitionforpf.org/2008/10/16/intermune-reports-japanese-regulatory-approval-of-pirfenidone-in-ipf/.

17. Susan Mayor, "Increasing Treatment of Idiopathic Pulmonary Fibrosis with Pirfenidone, European Survey Shows," *Medical News Today*, last modified December 6, 2012, accessed April 21, 2015, http://www.medicalnewstoday.com/articles/253656.php.

18. Alexander Tabarrok and Daniel Klein, "Reform Options," FDAReview.org, accessed April 19, 2015, http://www.fdareview.org/reform.shtml.

19. Paul Howard and Yevgeniy Feyman, "If a Drug Is Good Enough for Europeans, It's Good Enough for Us," *Health Affairs*, February 14, 2014, accessed April 20, 2015, http://healthaffairs.org/blog/2014/02/14/if-a-drug-is-good-enough-for-europeans-its-good-enough-for-us/.

20. Joseph A. DiMasi, Christopher-Paul Milne, and Alex Tabarrok, "An FDA Report Card: Wide Variance in Performance Found among Agency's Drug Review Divisions," Manhattan Institute, no. 7 (2014): 4, accessed April 27, 2015, http://www.manhattan-institute.org/pdf/fda_07.pdf.

21. Sam Kazman, "Drug Approvals and Deadly Delays," *Journal of American Surgeons* 15, no. 4 (2010): 102, accessed April 26, 2015, http://www.jpands.org/vol15no4/kazman.pdf.

22. Ibid., 102.

23. Howard and Feyman, "If a Drug Is Good Enough for Europeans, It's Good Enough for Us."

24. Henry I. Miller, "A Grieving Mother Acts, While the FDA Dithers," *Forbes*, May 21, 2014, accessed April 28, 2015, http://www.forbes.com/sites/henrymiller/2014/05/21/3230/.

25. Jonel Aleccia, "Vaccine Run: Grieving Mom Heads to Canada for Lifesaving Shots," *NBC News*, May 16, 2014, accessed April 27, 2015, http://www.nbcnews.com/health/health-news/vaccine-run-grieving-mom-heads-canada-lifesaving-shots-n106646.

26. Miller, "A Grieving Mother Acts, While the FDA Dithers."

27. US Food and Drug Administration, "FDA Approves a Second Vaccine to Prevent Serogroup B Meningococcal Disease," news release, January 23, 2015, accessed March 21, 2015, http://www.fda.gov/NewsEvents/Newsroom/PressAnnouncements/ucm431370.htm.

28. Andrew von Eschenbach and Ralph Hall, "FDA Approvals Are a Matter of Life and Death," *Wall Street Journal*, June 17, 2012, accessed February 14, 2015, http://www.wsj.com/articles/SB10001424052702303753904577454163076760768.

29. Peter Huber and Paul Howard, "Unlocking the Code of Health: Bridging the Gap Between Precision Medicine and FDA Regulation," *Project FDA Report* 8 (2015), accessed April 9, 2015, http://www.manhattan-institute.org/pdf/fda_08.pdf.

30. Peter Huber, "Patient, Heal Thyself," *City Journal* (Winter 2015), accessed March 29, 2015, http://www.city-journal.org/2015/25_1_cell-therapies.html.

31. Huber and Howard, "Unlocking the Code of Health."

32. FDA Checkup: Drug Development and Manufacturing Challenges: Hearing Before the Committee on Oversight and Government Reform, Subcommittee on Energy Policy, Health Care and Entitlements, House of Representatives, 113th Cong. (2013) (Testimony of Peter Huber).

33. "Exceptional Responders Initiative: Questions and Answers," National Cancer Institute, last modified March 23, 2015, accessed April 26, 2015, http://www.cancer.gov/news-events/press-releases/2014/exceptionalrespondersqanda.

34. Jim Epstein, "A Miracle Drug Cured Ed Levitt of Stage IV Lung Cancer. Then the FDA Withdrew It from the Market," *Reason*, December 3, 2013, accessed April 26, 2015, http://reason.com/blog/2013/12/03/a-miracle-drug-cured-ed-levitt-of-stage.

35. Mary A. Malarkey to Christopher J. Centeno, US Food and Drug Administration, July 25, 2008, accessed April 2, 2015, http://www.fda.gov/BiologicsBloodVaccines/GuidanceComplianceRegulatoryInformation/ComplianceActivities/Enforcement/UntitledLetters/ucm091991.htm.

36. "FDA: Your Body Is a Drug and We Want to Regulate It," Regenexx, February 2, 2012, accessed May 9, 2015, http://www.regenexx.com/2012/02/fda-your-body-is-a-drug-and-we-want-to-regulate-it/.

37. David Cyranoski, "FDA's Claims over Stem Cells Upheld," *Nature*, July 27, 2012, accessed May 19, 2015, http://www.nature.com/news/fda-s-claims-over-stem-cells-upheld-1.11082.

38. Karen Weintraub, "A 3-D-Printed Implant Saves Lives," *Technology Review*, April

30, 2015, accessed May 10, 2015, http://www.technologyreview.com/news/537166/a
-3-d-printed-implant-saves-lives/.

39. "New Study Shows How Babies' Lives Were Saved by 3D Printing," C. S. Mott Children's Hospital, April 29, 2015, accessed May 10, 2015, http://www.mottchildren.org/news/archive/201504/3dprinting.

## CHAPTER 9: IF YOU HAVE THE RIGHT TO DIE, YOU SHOULD HAVE THE RIGHT TO TRY

1. *Cruzan v. Director, Missouri Department of Health*, 497 U.S. 261, (1990).

2. *United States v. Rutherford*, 442 U.S. 544 (1979).

3. US Department of Health, Education, and Welfare, Food and Drug Administration, "Laetrile: The Commissioner's Decision," 77-3056 (HEW Publication), accessed May 11, 2015, http://www.cancertreatmentwatch.org/q/laetrile/commissioner.pdf.

4. US Food and Drug Administration, "Lengthy Jail Sentence for Vendor of Laetrile—A Quack Medication to Treat Cancer Patients," news release, June 22, 2004, accessed May 20, 2015, http://www.fda.gov/NewsEvents/Newsroom/PressAnnouncements/2004/ucm108314.htm.

5. "Laetrile/Amygdalin (PDQ®)," National Cancer Institute, last modified March 31, 2015, accessed April 12, 2015, http://www.cancer.gov/about-cancer/treatment/cam/patient/laetrile-pdq#section/all.

6. "How to Become a New Patient," Oasis of Hope, accessed March 23, 2015, http://www.oasisofhope.com/become_a_patient.php.

7. *Abigail Alliance v. von Eschenbach*, 495 F.3d 695 (D.C. Cir. 2007).

8. Ibid. at 714 (Rogers, J., dissenting).

9. Eugene Volokh, "Medical Self-Defense, Prohibited Experimental Therapies, and Payment for Organs," *Harvard Law Review* 120 (2007): 1813.

10. Ed Silverman, "Congressional Lawmakers Introduce a Right to Try Bill for Desperate Patients," *Wall Street Journal*, July 14, 2015, accessed July 15, 2015, http://blogs.wsj.com/pharmalot/2015/07/14/congressional-lawmakers-introduce-a-right-to-try-bill-for-desperate-patients/.

## AFTERWORD

1. Caroline Chen and Danielle Burger, "Sarepta CEO Quits; Successor Pledges to Work Better with FDA," *Bloomberg Business*, March 31, 2015, accessed June 6, 2015, http://www.bloomberg.com/news/articles/2015-04-01/duchenne-biotech-firm-sarepta-s-ceo-chris-garabedian-resigns.

2. "Sarepta Therapeutics Completes NDA Submission to FDA for Eteplirsen for the Treatment of Duchenne Muscular Dystrophy Amenable to Exon 51 Skipping," Sarepta Therapeutics, June 29, 2015 accessed July 3, 2015, http://investorrelations.sarepta.com/phoenix.zhtml?c=64231&p=irol-newsArticle&ID=2063150.

3. "Right to Try Stories: Diego Morris," Goldwater Institute, November 30, 2014, accessed December 12, 2015, http://goldwaterinstitute.org/en/work/topics/healthcare/right-to-try/right-to-try-life-stories-diego-morris/.

4. Saerom Yoo, "Cancer Survivor, 14, Advocates for Right to Try Bill," *Statesman Journal*, February 26, 2015, accessed June 6, 2015, http://www.statesmanjournal.com/story/news/health/2015/02/26/cancer-survivor-advocates-right-try-bill/24095681/.

5. "Oregon House Votes 59–0: Passes Right to Try Act to Effectively Nullify Some FDA Restrictions on Terminally-Ill," Tenth Amendment Center, April 8, 2015, accessed May 30, 2015, http://blog.tenthamendmentcenter.com/2015/04/oregon-house-votes-59-0-passes-right-to-try-act-to-effectively-nullify-some-fda-restrictions-on-terminally-ill/.

6. "What Are the Key Statistics about Osteosarcoma?" American Cancer Society, last modified January 6, 2015, accessed May 22, 2015, http://www.cancer.org/cancer/osteosarcoma/detailedguide/osteosarcoma-key-statistics.

7. Andrew Pollack, "Races for a Cure, Straight from the Heart," *New York Times*, May 27, 2001, accessed January 18, 2015, http://www.nytimes.com/2001/05/27/business/races-for-a-cure-straight-from-the-heart.html.

# Index

# About the Author

———

Darcy Olsen is the founder of Generation Justice, which champions constitutional protections for infants and children in foster care. She is also the former president and CEO of the Goldwater Institute, a leading national policy and litigation organization that has changed more than two hundred laws nationwide over the last several years. The group is leading the national campaign to pass Right to Try laws.